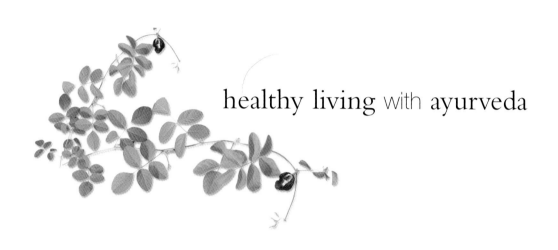

healthy living with ayurveda

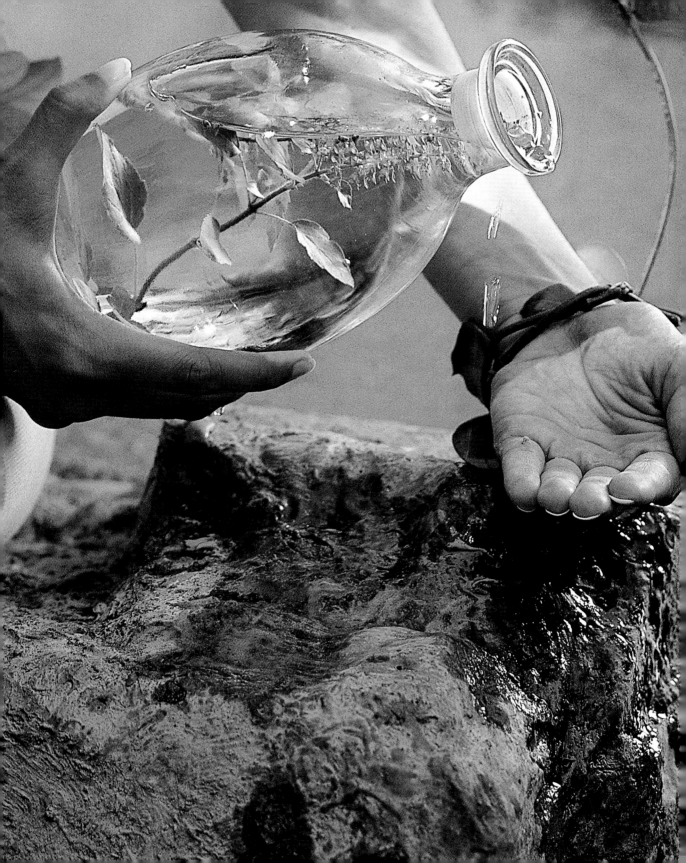

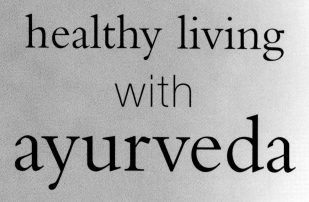

healthy living
with
ayurveda

Anuradha Singh

Lustre Press
Roli Books

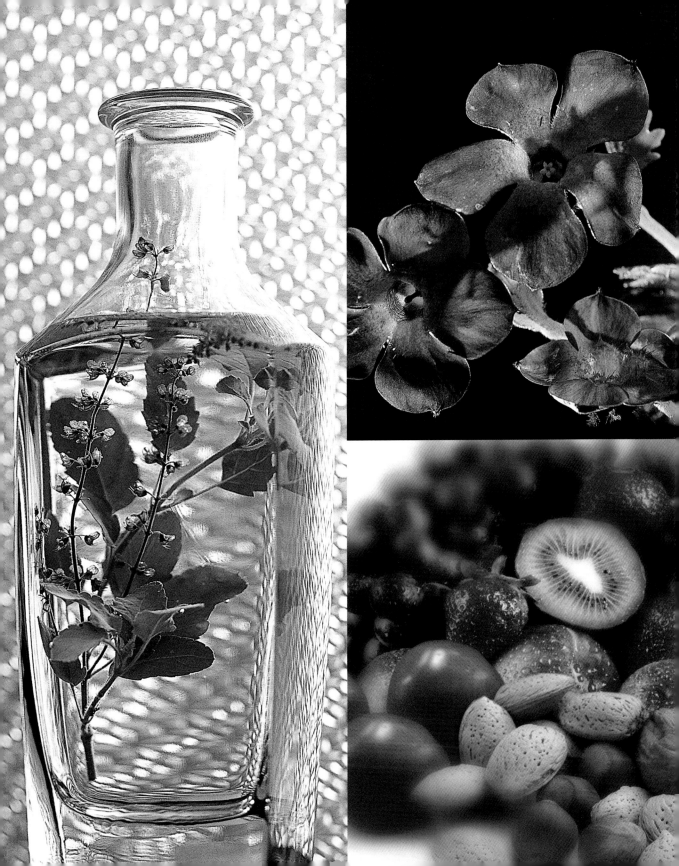

acknowledgements

*I would like to give my special thanks to
Vaidya Ramesh Nanal from Bombay.
I have made use of his expertise, through personal
communication and through his writings on Ayurveda.
However, all errors in this effort remain my responsibility.
I want to thank Dr Pushpjeet Phadke for encouraging me to write this
book. I also thank her for her unmatched, euphoric trust in my
abilities to communicate a difficult subject in an easy way.
I am indebted to Mayas and Apurva for making perceptive comments
and invaluable criticism. My indebtedness to Navjyoti remains beyond
words. His support and advice made this book possible.*

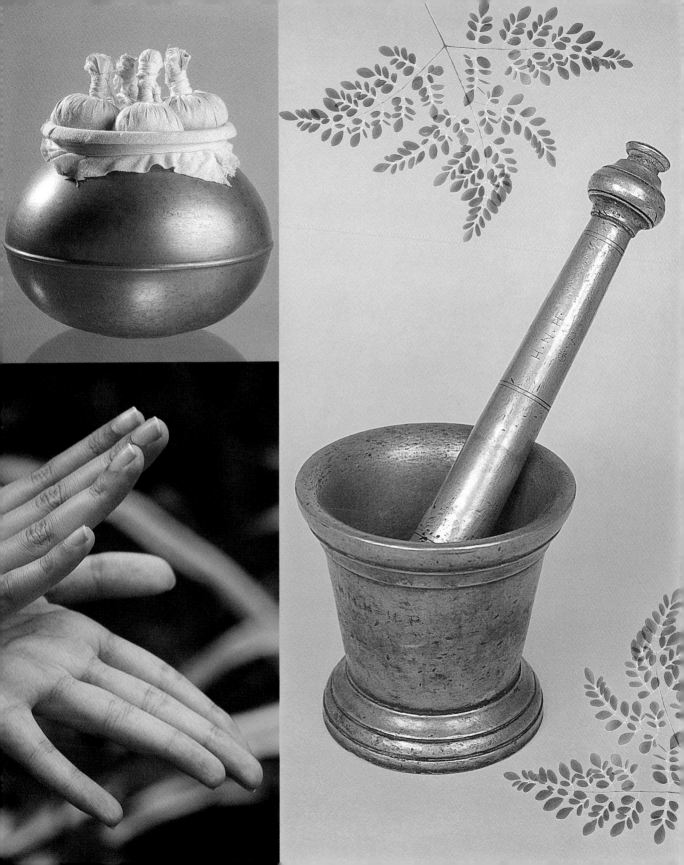

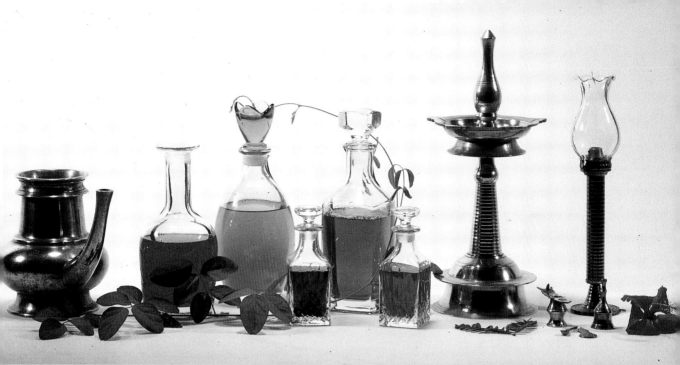

contents

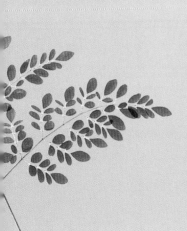

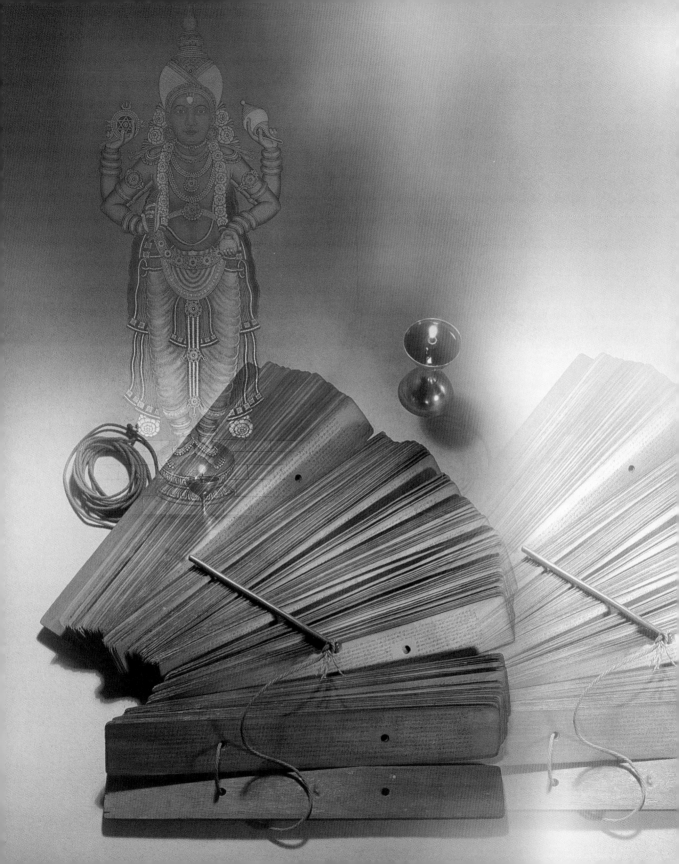

understanding
ayurveda
~

Rationale, Basic Principles and
Concepts, *Prakriti* Analysis

Ayurveda is a way of life. Familiarity with Ayurveda equips one for intelligent living. It is a system of knowledge that makes possible a fuller, more contented life. The primary subject matter of Ayurveda is life, or *ayus*. Life is a locus of experience (*anubhava*), action (*prayatna*) and disposition (*samskara*).

Any living organism is different from inanimate entities because it is infused with the property of *experience*. Experience triggers action. Experiences and actions are differentially determined by dispositions that characterize the organism; otherwise all living beings will be identical. It is the uniqueness and individuality of each living being that is denoted by *ayus* (often translated as life-span). *Ayus* refers to 'personhood', a capacity that remains constant between birth and death, a capacity that helps us navigate through ceaseless changes that invigorate or afflict living beings throughout a life span. It is the upkeep of this capacity which is the purpose of Ayurveda, or the science of *Ayus*.

The basic concepts of Ayurveda are derived from understanding *ayus* in human beings. A living person is not individual in the sense of being indivisible. A person is a compound of many aspects. Each person comprises of (1) body or *sarira*, (2) sense organs or *indriya*, (3) heart-mind or *manas*, and (4) self or *atman*. The body and sense organs are material, whereas the heart-mind and self are incorporeal. Experienced 'stream of consciousness' necessarily requires heart-mind, otherwise all experiences will clutter into a single conscious moment. Without the vehicle of the body and sense organs, neither is experience evidenced, nor the richness of experience accounted for. Personhood or *ayus* thus is a multi-entity cohesive compound.

Ayurveda is a science of the 'experienced' and 'felt' body and not merely the anatomical/chemical body. Matter, which alone constitutes the body, is accessible through the apparatuses of sense organs. There are five outer sensory apparatuses: visual (sight), tactile (touch), auditory (sound), gustatory (taste) and olfactory (smell). The sixth sensory apparatus, the heart-mind (*manas*), is an internal sense organ which makes available previous memories of experience.

If we look at the array of qualities given to us by sensory apparatuses, we will notice that each of these sense organs yields one special quality among others which are not accessed by other sense organs. Smell cannot be touched or seen. Taste cannot be heard or touched. Sound cannot be seen or smelt. Touch cannot be heard or tasted. Sight cannot be tasted or smelt. These are *special qualities* or secondary qualities which are given by one sense organ alone. Besides these qualities, there are

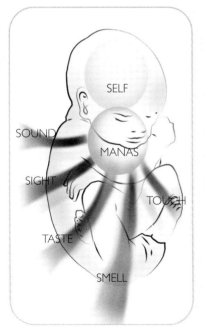

Person: A Compound of Self, *Manas,* Sense organs and Body

Self: The self explains the unity and continuity of experience in a person. It is a seat of consciousness, which is difficult to account for only on the basis of bodily processes.

Manas: *Manas* is required to explain the serialization of experience as a stream of conscious events in person. It is the missing link between the sense organs with the self and between a previous state of self and a new state of self. It distributes bodily, sensory and dispositional elements into a unified state of experience. It is an internal sense organ.

Sense organs: Sense organs are required to understand the experience of perception. They are the windows to the world of experience.

Body: The motor activity of a person is regulated by the body. Self, *manas* and sensory apparatuses work in conjuction with the body. A person perishes when the body dies.

other qualities, called the general qualities or primary qualities of matter that are given by two sense organs and can be recognized independently through touch and sight. For example, the 'number' of objects can be counted by touching and seeing, and the 'size' of objects can be known by touching and seeing.

Ayurveda is the science of experiential matter and not just of the experiential body

Sensory reality is phantasmic in character. Words, colours, textures, odours and tastes are phantasmic disclosures of reality. Specialized sensory apparatuses can work without fail because each of these five special qualities has a real material substrate. Material reality itself has to be such that these qualities can be experientially disclosed in an ordered way. If these qualities are authentic, their five exclusive material substrates are to be taken as real. These material substrates are called *panca mahabhuta*s (five grand stems of phantasm) and are commonly known as five elements. Whatever be the atomic and sub-atomic composition of matter, matter is finally structured in five elemental forms so that it remains amenable to sensation.

Ayurveda deals with sensory matter which is five-fold. Translations of elements as air, water, fire, earth and ether are a little misleading given their common use. They have to be conceived as formations of matter that are capable of holding sound, touch, vision, taste and smell. Sensory matter thus is of five kinds: *akasa* (ether) as a substrate of sound, *vayu* (air)

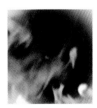 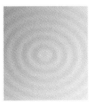 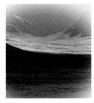 

~

There was a bright young boy who enrolled himself with an accomplished Ayurvedic teacher to master the science of Ayurveda. He was quick to learn every lesson the teacher gave him. Soon he had learnt all the texts of Ayurveda and its related arts and sciences. His talent earned him the respect and adulation of all. But he was impatient. Having learnt every lesson the teacher had to offer, he requested the teacher to graduate him so that he could practice Ayurveda. He was eager to apply his knowledge to cure the sick. The teacher, on learning of his desire, told him if he could answer a question satisfactorily he could graduate. The teacher asked him to bring a substance that had no medicinal property. The young boy, the epitome of confidence, told the teacher that he would fetch such a substance in an hours' time. He immediately set out to collect and bring back such a substance. Keen observer that he was, he would pick the most obscure of substances from the wayside, but upon examination would find it of some medicinal use. He wandered around inspecting all types of substances. Days, months and years passed by but he could not locate such a substance. After years of search, crestfallen, he returned empty-handed to his teacher and confessed 'I could not find any substance that has no medicinal property.' Gladdened by the sincere effort of the student the teacher gave him a last lesson. 'There is no substance in the universe that has no medicinal value. Having examined so many substances and their medicinal use, you have truly excelled as student and are now fully equipped to practice on your own.'

~

as a substrate of touch, *tejas* (fire) as a substrate of vision, *apa* (water) as a substrate of taste and *prithvi* (earth) as a substrate of smell. When matter goes into the body by way of food, breath or sensation it undergoes various operations. These operations need to be grasped to understand the nature of the influx-outflux matrix of matter in the body.

According to Ayurveda, there are three felt functions that are operative in the body. These are: *vata* (mover), *pitta* (transformer) and *kapha* (binder). Matter *moves* in the body; it is *transformed* in the body; it is *bound* in the body. These are the *three vehicles of change* in the body. They are commonly known as the three humours. These functions are a continuous process and they are diversely performed in an intricate material complex of the body. Body matter is *moved* through millions of channels in the body; body matter is variedly *transformed* into useful forms on several occasions; such transformed matter is *bound* at the appropriate place and bound matter is *unbound* to be moved out for excretion along with unused matter. These three vehicles are made out of matter and are a qualitative embodiment of material activity. They are vitalities in matter that characterize any changes in the body. They can be inferred from felt signatures in body. One of the ingenious features of Ayurvedic thinking is to sense, intuit, recognize and understand operations of these vitalities or vehicles of change. Influx-outflux is understood using these active forces. When the mover, transformer and binder functions are in balance the body is healthy. When they are vitiated, the body is imbalanced and ill. The body then needs restoration

Body Influx-outflux	
Intake	Output
Sensations	*Experience*
	Action
Dispositions	*Exhalation*
	Urine
	Feces
Inhalation	*Sweat*
	Mucus / Saliva
Food	*Tears*
	Earwax
Skin Absorption	*Hair*
	Nails

and corrective measures. Ayurveda defines disease as an imbalance (*vikriti*) of these vitalities, otherwise called *doshas* (fault-prone vitalities).

Each body is constitutionally disposed towards the over-performance or under performance of these functions individually or in combination. Otherwise there is no reason for all bodies not to be same. Understanding body types based on recognition of natural preponderance of these functions is essential to determining the *prakriti* (constitution) of a person. Such base constitutions of the body and root functional tendencies of the body usually do not change over a lifetime. It is because different bodies have different constitutions that the influx and outflux of the same matter is handled differently. The state of health and vulnerability towards disease differs as well. Understanding the root constitution of the body helps understand the character of matter passing through the body and the possibility of deviant development.

These vitalities operate on the material frame of the body. The body, *sarira* (literally, that which is disposed to decay), is made up of nine types

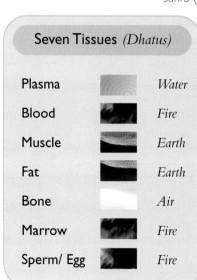

Seven Tissues *(Dhatus)*

Plasma		*Water*
Blood		*Fire*
Muscle		*Earth*
Fat		*Earth*
Bone		*Air*
Marrow		*Fire*
Sperm/ Egg		*Fire*

of tissues that are called *dhatus* (stems). These tissues are the matter cast into a form that makes a steady frame for the body. In spite of stability, the frame constantly changes, remaking itself and expelling worn out tissue. Food (*ahara*) is transformed into these tissues, moved to suitable places and appropriately bound. Similarly, decaying tissues are transformed, unbound and moved for excretion. Waste matter that is excreted is called *mala* (waste). *Mala* is not only made up of decaying tissues but also mal-transformed and un-transformed matter.

Intake to excretion path is marked by multiple systems of channels in the body. Out of the system of 15 channels, some connect the world outside the body with the world inside the body. Seven such channels are of – respiration, food, sperm/ovum, urine, feces, sweat and menstrual fluids. Seven channels in which matter moves are internal to body. These carry seven basic tissue types through the body in various stages of their transformation. One internal channel is meant for the motion of the heart-mind (*manas*). This is a neuronal channel in which the movement of *manas* leads to cogitation and other qualities of self (*atman*). Besides these channels that carry materials there are five openings of sense organs connected with the heart-mind channel on the one side and the external world on the other side. Obstruction of these channels leads to or is caused by malfunctioning of the body.

The material signs of malfunctioning and the seeds of disease lie in the accumulation or retention of *ama*, which is waste or unnecessary matter in the body. *Ama* is the presence of undigested food and toxic material intake in the body. All externally induced diseases are eventually

Channels of Breath	System of Channels	Channels of Bone Tissues
Channels of Water		Channels of Marrow
Channels of Food	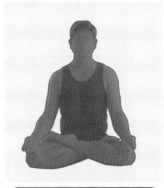	Channels of Sperm/Ovum
Channels of Nutritive Fluids		Channels of Urine
Channels of Blood		Channels of Feces
Channels of Muscle Tissues		Channels of Sweat
Channels of Fat Tissues	Channels of *Manas*	Channels of Menstrual Fluid

16

produced by *ama*. The absence of *ama* is a sign of well being which shows in the glow that radiates out of a healthy person. The opposite of *ama*, the vitalizing material formation responsible for this glow is called *ojas*. Abundance of *ojas* expresses itself by exuding strength, clarity and a focus of mind and body.

All substantial formations have a role in the construction and upkeep of a human being. Evolution itself is the experimentation of substances to create possible and plausible combinations. Earth, water, fire, air and ether mixed, morphed and stabilized into variegated material forms. At any evolutionary stage, natural, material and organic formations that have arrived through a fertile and chequered course of evolution have contributed to the evolution of a higher stage. Fecundity of life forms as well as inanimate-forms is related to man through the unity of the evolutionary process. No wonder that there is no substance that is of no medicinal use to man.

Today various naturally evolved substances are sufficient to correct internal malfunctioning. Minerals, herbs and animals constitute a grand depository worthy of an adequate diet, as well as for medical purposes. Elements of this depository are in fact collectively responsible for the constitution and upkeep of a person. For any need, we only have to realize the appropriate intake of one or another natural product. Reasoning with the selection of natural products for dietary and medicinal purposes is another important aspect of Ayurveda.

Reasoning with Sensate Matter

Ayurveda deals with those aspects of matter that are readily given to sensation and experience. Sensate matter is an aspect of matter with sensory qualities; it is matter as given in experience and not matter that exists independent of experience. Ayurveda has evolved a reasoning about the action of matter, especially with respect to the body, with sensory and other qualities. It is important to understand this aspect of Ayurvedic reasoning to fully live with the categories and concepts of Ayurveda.

Apart from qualities that are given by each sense organ and the general qualities of matter which are also sensed by sensory apparatuses, there are *'actional' qualities of matter*. These actional qualities represent the causative potential of material substances. Material substances act and actional qualities qualify material substances for their action. For example, 'hot' and 'cold' are such actional qualities of substances. They are not simply thermodynamic properties. Yogurt is 'hot' in its nature; it has the power to heat up the stomach when consumed. On churning the yogurt, physical heat is added to it, but the resultant buttermilk is 'cold' in its nature. Consuming buttermilk cools the stomach. Thus 'hot' and 'cold' attributes of substances do not really characterize *physical heat* but *sensate heat*. 'Hot' and 'cold' are simple *experienced attributes* that are given to human experience by the heart-mind with the help of the other sense organs. They characterize the potential effect of a material substance when consumed.

Causal Reasoning in Ayurveda

The body is characterized in Ayurveda in accordance with vital functions — mover/transformer/binder — which can be vitiated. So, a diet or drugs with balance-inducing actional qualities can correctively act on these functions alone and help restore normalcy. Actional qualities are thus

According to Ayurveda there are ten pairs of opposing actional qualities (twenty in all), that qualify substances for their causative potential.

heavy *guru*	**light** *laghu*
cold *sita*	**hot** *usna*
unctuous *snigdha*	**dry** *ruksa*
slow *manda*	**acute** *tiksna*
stable *sthira*	**mobile** *sara*
soft *mrdu*	**hard** *kathina*
clear *visada*	**slimy** *picchila*
dense *sandra*	**fluid** *drava*
smooth *slaksna*	**rough** *khara*
subtle *suksma*	**coarse** *sthula*

These sensate qualities are complex because they are not directly correlated with corresponding physical qualities. Though in terms of sensations they are simple, they are not given to experience by any particular external sense organ. Tactile sensory apparatus neither senses a 'hot' substance as hot, nor is the 'hot' nature explained by the physical heat capacity. Chilli is 'hot' in nature but on touching it we do not get any sensation of physical heat. 'Hot' nature perhaps embodies the effect material substance can have on the body. Similarly, 'heavy' and 'light' qualities are not just the physical weight or density of material substances. Pistachios are 'heavy' even when only a few are eaten, whereas puffed rice is 'light' even when consumed in large quantities.

directly related to imbalances of vital functions (*doshas*). Vital functions themselves are characterized by actional qualities:

Mover/Ether, Air

Vata: Dry, cold, light, rough, mobile, clear, subtle.
Respiration; circulation; excretion; movement; sexual activity brain activity; feeling; sensation; foetus growth.

Transformer/Fire

Pitta: Unctuous, hot, light, acute, fluid, free flowing.
Vision; body heat; digestion; hunger; lustre of body; vigour; cheerfulness; cognition.

Binder/ Earth, Water

Kapha: unctuous, cold, heavy, slow, stable, slimy, smooth, soft, dense.
Structure of body; potency; heaviness; firmness; strength; restraint; forbearance.

Mover and Transformer are light and only Binder is heavy. Mover and Binder are cold and only Transformer is hot. Transformer and Binder are unctuous (moist and oily) and only Mover is dry.

The vital principles are peculiar configurations of actional qualities. Of these twenty qualities, elementary Ayurvedic reasoning employs the first six extensively. This is because the first six characterize the body's vital functions uniquely, as well as in mutual comparison, rather neatly.

There are three causal principles used in Ayurveda for altering the qualitative state of the body:

1. The quality in the body that is desired to be changed increases with the infusion of same quality substance, and;

2. The quality in the body that is desired to be changed decreases with the infusion of opposite quality substance.
   Using these principles, vital functions in the body can be differentially accentuated, repressed or altered in any desired way by the intake of an appropriately designed diet or drug. There is a third causal principle used in Ayurveda for altering the qualitative state of the body.

3. The quality of a substance can undergo change when brought into contact with fire.
   As a principle, this is used to prepare the appropriate diet or drug. Sensate matter can be transformed in its sensory qualities with the application of fire, much like the colour of an unbaked pot is affected by baking.

Bodies as unique constitutions

For a fuller grasp of the causal reasoning in Ayurveda it is important to know the root disposition of the body in terms of vital functions. Each body is unique in its constitution. However, there are seven basic types of prominent constitutions in terms of the root tendency of a body towards vital functions. These seven constitutions, called *prakrti,* are –

dominant binder; dominant transformer; dominant mover; dominant binder-transformer; dominant transformer-mover; dominant mover-binder, and; balanced binder-transformer-mover. It is important to know the constitution of any particular body before the causal effect of a particular diet/drug can be worked out for that person. Ayurvedic analysis begins with determining the constitution (or root disposition) of a particular body. It is only after such an analysis that any nurturing, preventive and curative regimen of diet/drug can be thought of for the person. Living with Ayurveda can truly start after determining one's constitution.

Know your constitution

We give below 28 different features of the body that typically differentiate the prominence of one of the three vital functions. Each person has all three vital functions. Even in a normal state, a person has at least one prominent vital function in comparison with the other vital functions. To determine your or anyone else's root constitution *(prakriti)*, just tick the feature options that match in each row. Count the number of times mover/transformer/binder options are selected through 28 rows. Depending on the number of mover, transformer and number of binder features selected, your constitution can be mechanically determined. It is always advisable to crosscheck the *prakriti* determined this way with a competent Ayurvedic physician.

With the results obtained after counting the features selected from the mover, transformer and binder columns, one can compare the count with the table below to roughly obtain a person's root constitution.

KNOW YOUR CONSTITUTION

Features	Mover *(vata)*	Transformer *(pitta)*	Binder *(kapha)*
Body Structure	Thin and slim physique.	Tall, medium, moderately developed physique.	Stout, big and well developed physique.
Chest	Narrow	Barrel Shaped	Square and well-formed
Bone Structure	Low, prominent bones.	Moderate bones, good muscles.	Heavy bones, tendency towards obesity.
Weight	Hard to gain and easy to lose.	Easy to gain and easy to lose.	Easy to gain and hard to lose.
Skin Texture	Thin, dry, cold, rough, cracked skin.	Warm, moist, skin often with moles and prone to acne.	White, oily, smooth and soft skin.
Hair Texture	Scanty, coarse, dry, wavy hair.	Fine, soft, red or gray hair often balding in early age.	Dark, thick, oily, lustrous hair.
Forehead Shape	Small forehead.	Medium sized forehead.	Broad forehead.
Face	Sharp features, masked appearance.	Gentle features, warm appearance.	Broad features.
Eyes	Small, often brown eyes.	Medium size, piercing eyes.	White, attractive, large eyes with thick eyelashes.
Lips	Thin, small dry lips.	Medium, soft, red lips.	Thick, moist lips.
Teeth & Gums	Irregular sized teeth, dark gums.	Medium sized teeth, spongy gums.	Shiny straight smooth teeth, pink gums.
Nails	Small, thin, dry nails.	Soft, pink, medium nails	Large, white nails.
Stools	Prone to constipation.	Regular.	Moderate.
Sweat	Scanty sweat.	Profuse.	Moderate cold sweat.

Features	Mover *(vata)*	Transformer *(pitta)*	Binder *(kapha)*
Appetite	Appetite is variable.	Strong appetite. Irritable if meal is missed.	Can skip meals easily.
Sexuality	Variable.	Hot and intense.	Warm and enduring.
Voice	Low, weak, hoarse voice.	High pitched, sharp voice.	Deep tone, pleasant voice.
Speech	Talkative, talk fast.	Convincing speech. Argumentative.	Slow, definite speech. Not very talkative.
Intellect	Quick, adaptable, indecisive mental. nature	Intelligent, critical mental nature.	Slow, steady, dull mental nature.
Memory	Good observation, but poor memory.	Sharp, clear memory.	Slow to take notice but will not forget easily.
Nature	Fearful, anxious.	Angry and irritable.	Calm, sentimental.
Sleep	Light, disturbed sleep. Tends towards insomnia.	Moderate sleep. Wakes up at the smallest sound.	Heavy sleep, difficulty in waking up.
Type of dreams	Flying, moving, restless in dreams.	Colorful (especially red), passionate.	Few, sentimental and romantic dreams.
Climatic Preference	Prefer warm climate, sunshine and moisture.	Prefer cool and well ventilated place.	Any climate is fine as long as it is not humid.
Financial matters	Spends money quickly.	Spends money on luxuries.	Saves money.
Tastes	Likes sweet, sour and salty tastes.	Likes sweets, bitter and astringent tastes.	Likes pungent, bitter and astringent tastes.
Tendency to Types of diseases	Nervous system diseases, pain, arthritis, mental disorders.	Fevers, infections and inflammatory diseases.	Respiratory system diseases.
Type of pulse	Rapid, irregular and weak pulse.	Strong, pulse.	Steady, rhythmic pulse.

YOUR CONSTITUTION

Mover Count	Transformer Count	Binder Count	Root Constitution
>20			Mover
	>20		Transformer
		>20	Binder
>12	>12		Mover-Transformer
	>12	>12	Transformer-Binder
>12		>12	Binder-Mover
8<…<12	8<…<12	8<…<12	Mover-Transformer-Binder

Once the typical root constitution of a person is determined, the basic tendencies of a person are known. Vulnerability to disease is identified, and receptivity to the diet/drugs required can be established. It becomes possible to accurately customize diet/drugs for a person. Vital functions wax and wane cyclically even through a day, a month and through seasons. Sensitivity towards and awareness of these changes can help manage the body well in terms of suitable regimen, diet and medication.

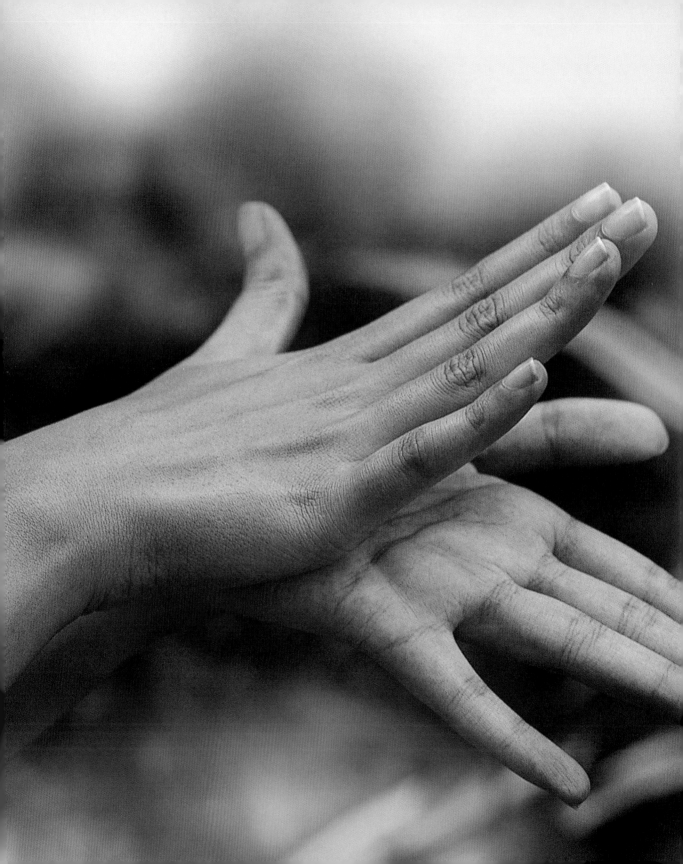

practicing the
ayurvedic way
~

Daily, Weekly, Monthly,

Seasonal and Epochal Practices

Living each day according to the specific requirements of one's body is crucial to living with Ayurveda. Knowledge of Ayurveda is relevant only when applied to day-to-day living, incorporated in lifestyle, proving effective in making choices beneficial for achieving optimal health. There are various external forces that are cyclically active in everyday situations. The body is susceptible to these forces and their understanding paves way for decisions regarding daily regimens to be followed.

Cyclic Regimens

The basic influence on the properties, interaction and efficacy of material substances comes from major cyclic material phenomena around us. Cyclic motions of the earth, sun and moon directly influence the behaviour of matter inside and outside the body. Thus, there are three basic cycles that are fundamental to our well being:

SLEEP–WAKING CYCLE: The earth's rotation around its axis creates this cycle. The daily regimen of a person is derived from this basic cycle. Intake and excretion cycles of the body are dependent on this cycle. The upkeep of normal body functions require daily cleansing.

MONTHLY CYCLE: The moon's revolution around the earth creates its waxing and waning cycle. The monthly regimen of a person is derived from this basic cycle. It also helps mark sections of the seasonal cycle. Special cleansing of the body for accumulated toxins is related to this cycle.

SEASONAL CYCLE: Because of the tilted earth's revolution around the sun, the north-south motion over a year creates this cycle. The seasonal regimen of a person is derived from this basic cycle. Seasonal variation, the susceptibility of the body to ordinary disease and preventive regimen depend on this cycle.

YEARLY CYCLE: The earth's repeated revolution around the sun creates this cycle. The yearly regimen of a person is derived from this basic cycle. Cleansing of toxins responsible for chronic abrasions of the body can be associated with this cycle.

Besides these four cycles, there are cycles that are related to civil and cultural practice.

WEEKLY CYCLE: This results from working and holiday cycles. The regimen of a person on weekdays and weekends changes because of these cycles. Holidays provide an opportunity to address neglected aspects of the upkeep of the body.

EPOCHAL CYCLE: This results from the physical ageing of a person. Age related regimen is derived from this basic cycle. Mechanisms for the rejuvenation of the body depend on this cycle.

When we look at the effect of these cycles on regimen, three concepts are important: the onset of the cycle, setting of the cycle and transition across cycles. Being mindful of such points of various cycles creates opportunities to undertake various Ayurvedic practices.

Daily Cycle

Waking up ~ Drinking Water in the Morning
Bowel Cleansing ~ Mouth and Teeth
Throat and Gargling ~ Nasal Passage ~ Ear ~ Eyes ~ Skin
Paste Massage ~ Exercise ~ Bath ~ Meditation ~ Breakfast
At the Office ~ Lunch ~ Evening ~ Dinner ~ Bed Time

Waking up

The body's biological clock is synchronized with the sun's natural clock. Sunrise does change with seasons, but the average time to wake up is between 4.00 am to 6.00 am, which is considered *brahma muhurata,* the time of the gods. It is also a time when the mover *(vata)* is dominant. The body at this time can absorb the subtleness of nature. It is also the time when *sattva gunas* (quintessence qualities) are dominant in nature. If the body gets tuned to waking up at this time, half the battle of beginning a good day is won. You wake up feeling light and calm at this time of the day. Usually binder *(kapha)* natured people get up the earliest; transformer *(pitta)* natured people wake up a little later, and; mover *(vata)* natured people wake up late. People with different constitutions tend to awaken when their constituent dominant vitalities are minimal in the morning.

It is advisable that one get up at the same time everyday. This is not only good for civic routines but also for the body. There could be occasional changes in this routine, but the attempt should be to come back to the consistent waking time.

Upon waking, if you wish, you can say a little prayer, or just remember the Almighty. This is the time to remember your indebtedness to the physical and spiritual world. The qualities of dawn create an apt occasion for this deed.

Drinking water in the morning

Splash water on the face and rinse the mouth after waking. This is a refreshing act that prepares you for a day ahead and marks switch from the night regime to the day regime. This washes away slumber leftover from sleeping.

After waking, one should drink water. Drink one or two glasses of water, or as much as one can comfortably drink. The water should be of normal temperature, neither hot nor cold. Drinking water helps in bowel movement, flushes out toxins from large intestine and helps in regulating evacuation of waste from the body. Liquids other than water stress the digestive system, which is undesirable first thing in the morning. Water directly helps in flushing of toxins through urination.

Drinking water is contraindicated if the abdomen feels distended, if the body is suffering from *vata* or *kapha* disease or after cleaning a wound

Vata dominant time to be awake
and alert 2 am - 7 pm.
Pitta dominant time to have the
main meal of the day 12 pm - 2 pm.
Kapha dominant time to
rest and sleep 6 pm - 10 pm.

After drinking water one should walk around for a while till the pressure is built for bladder and bowel cleansing. It is ideal to go for evacuation everyday at the same time.

Bowel cleansing

Not having a regular bowel movement has a direct effect on one's physical and psychological well being. The body's rhythms are synchronized with those in nature. At night the body is occupied with restructuring, recouping, nurturing and correcting itself. When the sun rises and internal fires *(agni)* become active, the body begins the absorption process. The waste created during the rest cycle is to be eliminated during the first active period of the body. If this waste is not evacuated, the body will carry it through the day, absorb its toxins and weaken itself. The feeling of heaviness, fatigue and depression may set in. One tends to feel light and relaxed, if the body has eliminated its night waste properly. Healthy bowel cleansing is a once in a day practice unlike bladder cleansing, which can happen 4 to 6 times a day. One has to take care that bowel cleansing remains a once or twice a day natural practice. This is a most significant activity for waste and toxin clearing from the system of person. Mental preoccupation hinders bowel cleansing, since the *prana vayu* (air connected with activities of the mind) is not free to help the *apana vayu* (air responsible for evacuation). When the mind is troubled, bodily functions are troubled. It is also useful to be observant of the evacuated faeces. If one spots any major deviation in regular bowel movements, one needs to pay attention for adjustment of the diet accordingly. These deviations are only indicative of imbalance in the body which if not corrected can become chronic problems.

Cleansing of the mouth and teeth

Traditionally, Indians used neem twigs *(Azadirachta indica)* or *babul (Acacia arabica)*, or liquorices for cleaning teeth and gums. Tooth powders made out of roasted almond shells and dried leaves of the above-mentioned herbs are also used for cleansing the teeth and the gums.

Modern day toothpastes are meant to clean the teeth, but generally have a sweet aftertaste that encourages bacterial growth in the mouth. Ayurveda strictly maintains that any teeth cleaner should have an astringent or pungent taste. A small change towards

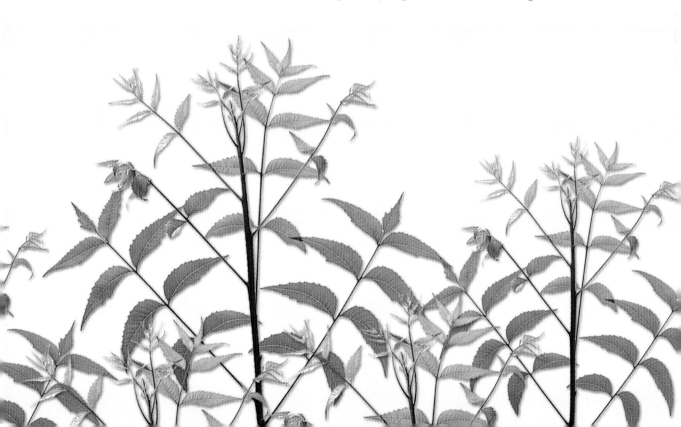

a more natural teeth cleaner can enhance oral hygiene. A soft twig crushed at one end can be chewed and used as a toothbrush to clean the teeth. Ayurvedic toothpastes are also available in the market.

Along with teeth cleaning, tongue cleaning has been given equal importance in Ayurveda. The appearance of the tongue is an important indication of what is going on inside the body. A white-coated tongue indicates the presence of excess mucus in the system; it also indicates improper digestion or presence of waste (*ama*) in the system. A yellowish tongue suggests to look for any bilious or transformer (*pitta*) imbalance in the liver or gallbladder. A bluish hue can be an indication of heart distress. A grayish tongue is a sign of vata imbalance or colon malfunctioning. All of these require immediate attention.

According to Ayurveda, the accumulation of waste at the root of the tongue subtly obstructs respiration and as a consequence gives rise to foul smelling breath. The tongue should be scraped regularly.

The tongue scraper was traditionally made of metals like gold, silver, tin or brass. Or simply, the twig used for brushing was also used for the purpose. Steel and bamboo tongue scrapers are available these days. To clean the tongue, one has to gently scrape the tongue from the back to the outer edges. Six to seven strokes are enough to clean the tongue. Thereafter the mouth is to be rinsed with water. Any accumulated binder (*kapha*) in the mouth and throat regions gets cleared this way. It not only cleans and freshens the mouth and breath; it sharpens the sense of taste. Keeping sense organs alert is important. The involuntary contraction of the stomach, which takes place at the time of scraping the tongue, prepares excreting boundaries and strengthens the muscles of the stomach. Clearing the mouth and nose through the day is important since the intake of breath and food for the upkeep of the body is routed through them.

Gargling

Gargling is considered equally important in maintaining oral hygiene. One can gargle with warm water, warm salted water or with triphala or liquorice powders added to plain warm water. Warm black tea also can be used for this purpose. It clears the throat and oral cavity, vitalizing them. Prolonged freshness of breath can be ensured this way.

Taking care of the nasal passage

Blow the nose once or twice and rinse the nostrils. A blocked nose needs to be taken seriously, as it can be symptomatic of potential disorders in the body leading to headaches, pain in the eyes or ears, sinus, or migraine to name a few. According to Ayurveda, as a routine, one should take few drops of sesame oil on the little finger and insert in each nostril and apply it on the inside. *Nasya,* as this act is called, is taken in other forms also like through medicated powders (which are sniffed), smoke or vapours.

Since the nose, according to Ayurveda, is actually a gateway to the brain, its care is of utmost important. 'Oileation' of the nasal passage not only imparts clarity and strength to sense organs of the eyes, ears and nose, it prevents hair loss, headaches, facial paralysis and tremors of the head. Ayurveda advises that if *nasya* is done regularly, afflictions of old age do not affect the mind.

Cleansing of the ears

One can apply a little sesame oil inside the ears. One or two drops can be directly poured in the ears. This keeps the mover *(vata)* balanced in ears. It not only sharpens the sense of hearing, it also prevents hearing loss, ringing in the ears and excessive formation of earwax. Furthermore, it provides tranquillity to the mind.

Focus on the eyes

Eyes are considered as the most important sense organ since they are windows to the outside world. Eyes are susceptible to binder *(kapha)* and transformer *(pitta)* imbalance, so the diet and the regimen should be such as to keep the eyes healthy. As a routine fill the mouth with water and then splash water gently on the eyes. Thereafter spit the water out. The best eyewash decoction is a *triphala* (three herbs, see page 147) solution, which can be prepared either by soaking it over night or by boiling it and then cooling and straining it, so that we have a clear water without any

Eyes are considered as
the most important sense
organ since they are windows
to the outside world

particles to wash the eyes. One can also dip the eyes and blink them in this decoction after putting it in an eyeglass.

Skin, massage and vital points

The skin is the largest human sense organ and is susceptible to mover *(vata)* imbalance. A morning massage *(abhyanga)*, if added to the daily routine, can be one of the most powerful healing activities. According to Ayurveda, dry skin becomes strong and resistant to any dysfunction with the application of oil. Similarly, the human body becomes strong and resistant to any disease. It also becomes resistant to exhaustion and exertion. Massage needs to be done on an empty stomach in the morning or preferably after 3 to 4 hours of consuming the afternoon meal. Massage should never be done on a full stomach.

As part of the daily routine, one can do self-massage. Massage the scalp, back of the neck, ear lobes (with thumbs and index fingers), temples, back and forth motion on arms, circular motion on joints, naval and abdomen and rounding it off with special attention to the hands and feet.

According to Ayurveda, massaging the feet has a direct effect on the eyes (both are governed by the fire element); regular massage of the feet promotes good eyesight, along with the benefits to the entire body. The soles of the feet have four important nerves which are connected to the head. When they are massaged, these nerves are stimulated, resulting in good eyesight and sound sleep. This connection can also be observed when one walks barefoot on morning grass full of dew. Such a walk is very refreshing for the eyes; it takes away excess heat from the eyes and has a calming effect.

Choice of the oils for massage

One has to ascertain one's constitution before choosing the oil for the body massage. For a head massage usually cooling oils are used. For the routine body massage, warming oils can be used.

The mover (*vata*) constitution is dry and cool; warm sesame oil is best suited for mover people. They can also use olive oil and almond oil. Essential oils like basil, cedar wood, musk and sage can also be used.

The skin of transformer (*pitta*) natured people requires cooling massage oils, as they are sensitive and are prone to eruptions or rashes. Coconut and sandalwood oil is best suited for those with transformer (*pitta*) constitution. They can also use sunflower oil. Essential oils like chamomile, cinnamon, rose and saffron can balance vitiated transformer (*pitta*) *dosha*.

The mover (*vata*) constitution is dry and cool; warm sesame oil is best suited for mover people. They can also use olive oil and almond oil. Essential oils like basil, cedar wood, musk and sage can also be used.

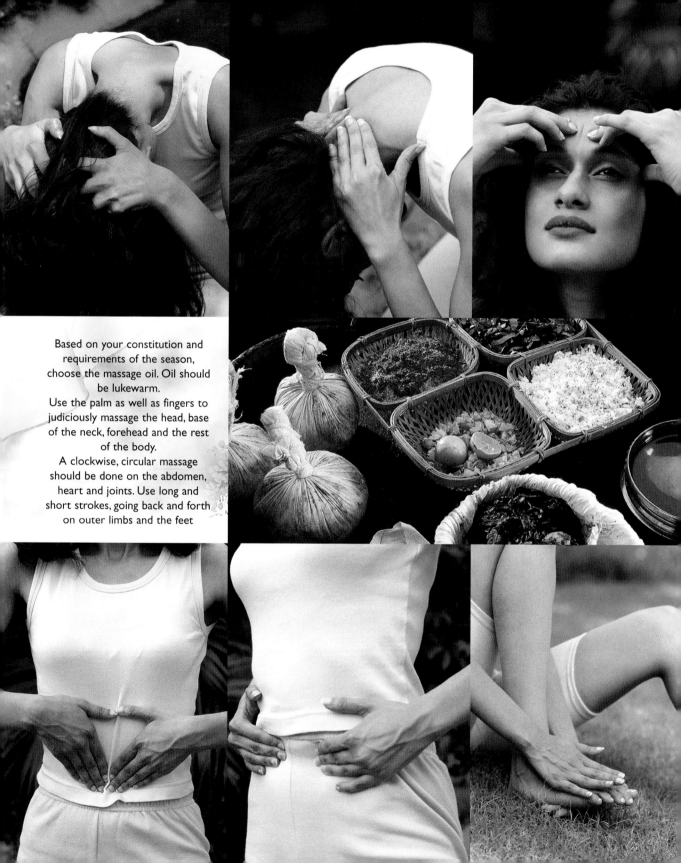

Based on your constitution and requirements of the season, choose the massage oil. Oil should be lukewarm.

Use the palm as well as fingers to judiciously massage the head, base of the neck, forehead and the rest of the body.

A clockwise, circular massage should be done on the abdomen, heart and joints. Use long and short strokes, going back and forth on outer limbs and the feet

Binder (*kapha*) natured people need little or no oil. The massage can be done with a little sesame or mustard oil or dry powders of calamus (*vaca*), dry ginger or black gram. The massage to the binder (*kapha*) people should be vigorous and with pressure. Essential oils like basil, camphor, lemon and frankincense can also be used.

Twice a week, one should also provide the body with the dry friction massage (*gharsana*). An invigorating dry rubbing of the body can be done with a soft bristle brush or with a soft towel.

Daily massage pacifies the mover (*vata*) and opens energy channels of the body. The pressure while doing massage not only improves circulation, it releases impurities of the body. The body absorbs the oil through its pores. The oil balances the mover (*vata*) and removes fatigue, weakness and roughness of the body, relaxes the nerves and calms the mind.

Massaging vital points (*marmas*)

The point at which the muscle tissues, veins, ligaments, bones and joints meet is called a *marma*. This is the point where the most concentration of airy (*pranika*) movement is found. While a full body massage is

The skin of transformer (*pitta*) natured people requires cooling massage oils, as they are sensitive and are prone to eruptions or rashes. Coconut and sandalwood oil is best suited for those with transformer (*pitta*) constitution. They can also use sunflower oil. Essential oils like chamomile, cinnamon, rose and saffron can balance vitiated transformer (*pitta dosha*).

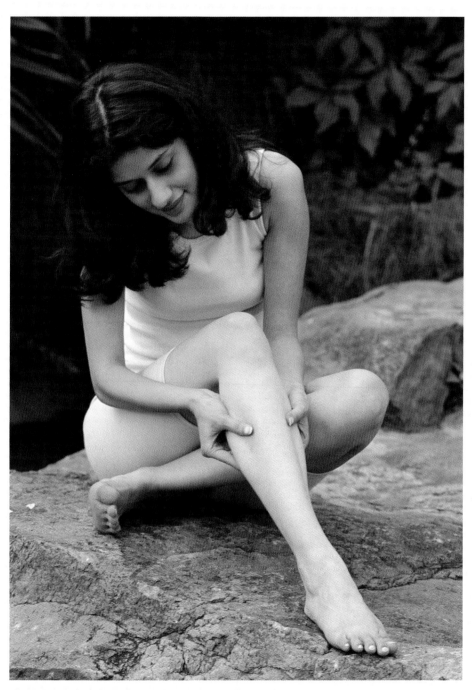

A full body massage is given utmost importance in Ayurveda. *Marmas* need to be given special attention when applying oil.

given utmost importance in Ayurveda, *marmas* need to be given special attention while applying oil or pressure. These *marmas* on the one hand sustain bodily vitalities and on the other, if injured can cause serious damage to the body, and can even result in death. However, a regular massage can stimulate the *marmas,* provide healing to the related body organs, cleanse and energize the internal body channels. Most Ayurvedic texts have mentioned 107 *marmas* in the body. In ancient times, the practical application of the knowledge of the *marmas* was done in the field of surgery, warfare and hunting. Its application in the upkeep of the body takes the form of *abhyanga* (massage), *lepam* (putting various herbal pastes), *pichu* (putting tamps on marmas), *dhara* (constant pouring of oil or milk or buttermilk on either the entire body or the specific body parts) and *sirobasti* (keeping the oil on the head, contained by a cap) for protective and curative treatments of the *marmas*.

Binder (*kapha*) natured people need little or no oil. The massage can be done with little sesame or mustard oil or dry powders of calamus (*vaca*), dry ginger or black gram. The massage to the binder (*kapha*) people should be vigorous and with pressure. Essential oils like basil, camphor, lemon and frankincense can also be used.

These treatments are specialized, but they are extremely effective in correcting any imbalance occurring in mind and body. However, for the purpose of everyday care of the body, ears, head and feet, remain the most important vital points according to

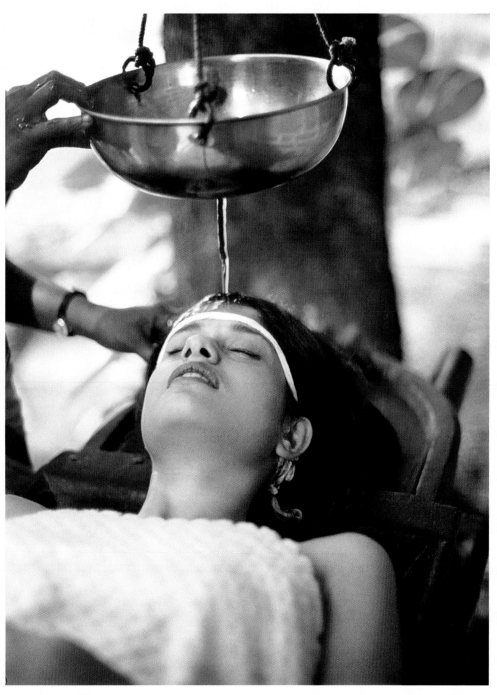

Preventive and curative treatment of the *marmas* include *dhara* (pouring of oil on specific body parts) and *sirobasi* (keeping oil on the head contained by a CP).

Ayurveda. Their oileation and proper massage go a long way in keeping the body healthy.

Paste massage (*ubtana*)

Traditionally and to this day, Indians have been using various herbs and ingredients used in household cooking for making pastes called *ubtanas* to smear on the body before bathing. This clears the residual oil from the body, cleans the pores and makes the skin soft, resistant to aberration and ageing. These pastes are made from various ingredients according to the season and skin types. *Ubtana* is handy, cost-effective and a unique cleanser after the oil massage and before bathing.

Generally, the paste is made with grains or legume flours with or without mixing in herbal powders. The paste *(ubtana)* can be dry or wet. For dry and rough skin, milk is added to the flour; otherwise rose water remains an ideal choice to make a wet paste. Turmeric powder *(haldi)* is considered an ideal choice of most of the Indian households to be put in their ubtana preparation along with the chosen flour. For all seasons and for all body types, green gram (whole *mung*) powder is considered a nourishing *ubtana*. However, for mover *(vata)* dominant skins, *urad, mung,* wheat and oats can be used. For transformer *(pitta)* dominant skins, chickpeas, barley, *urad* and wheat; for binder *(kapha)* dominant skins, *mung,* red lentil, millet and barley can be used for making an *ubtana*. For removing the excess oil, dry powder can be used on the body making the upward movements. However, while removing the powder, one needs to make downward movements to cleanse the body followed by a refreshing bath.

Exercise and Yoga

Some active exercises or yoga postures (for example, *surya namaskara* or sun salutations) should be part of everyday regimen as it aims at building strength and muscular movement for overall fitness. According to Ayurveda, it should be done on an empty stomach and according to the requirement of one's body. Done judiciously, it increases immunity, makes the body light, increases digestive powers and reduces the body's fats. Exercise is contra-indicated for excessively mover (*vata*) people, or when thirsty, hungry or after sexual activity, after travelling or heavy labour.

Mover (*vata*)

These people are involved with activities that require bursts of energy and speed like dance, ballet, aerobics and table tennis. However, they need less exercise; they can do slow duration, low-impact exercises like walking, cycling, swimming or yoga

Transformer (*pitta*)

These people are good at competitive sports that require stamina and enduring strength like weightlifting, tennis, track and field etc. However, they need to balance their competitive spirit with cooling sports like golf, cycling, swimming etc.

Binder (*kapha*)

These people are good at long term, enduring skills like archery, baseball, golf etc., since their grounded nature and stability make them perform well under pressure. However, they need to do more of vigorous exercises like running, rowing, and high impact aerobics.

Bathing

According to Ayurveda, bathing is a daily ritual. It is purifying and life-giving. It stimulates the body and removes fatigue, sweat and dirt. It is an excellent remedy for enhancing the *ojas,* the essence of all *dhatus,* the tissue elements. The choice of water is made according to season and the *prakriti* of the person. Mover (*vata*) people can have a warm water bath; transformer (*pitta*) people need cold water, and binder (*kapha*) people require hot water for bathing themselves. A bath is not just a great cleanser, it is refreshing too, as it takes away exhaustion and heaviness. A bath soothes the body and stimulates the mind and the senses.

Pranayama and Meditation

In the busy routine of our everyday lives, pausing to connect to one's higher self requires just a little orientation. After bathing, if one can add *pranayama* and meditation in the daily routine, the results can be seen, both in the gross and the subtle bodies. *Pranayama* is the art of observing and controlling the vital breath. It is deeply therapeutic, clearing all channels and making the body vibrantly healthy. Meditation is like a bath for the mind. It can lead to a clearer and deeper knowledge of oneself. For details of *pranayama* and meditation techniques and methods one can get information from the books specializing on the topic. However, it is best to learn the actual practices and their finer nuances under the supervision of a very learned and experienced teacher.

Natural urges

Ayurveda classifies natural desires, urges or dispositions which we are confronted with in two categories, (1) Suppressible urges and (2) Non suppressible urges. Suppressible natural urges include: malicious thoughts, speech and action, gred, anger, fear and violence.

Happiness and a virtuous life are the consequences of transcending the suppressible urges. People, who want to adopt the desirable practices but are addicted to unwholesome practices, are advised to give up the undesirable practices slowly. According to Ayurveda such a transition should come very gradually so that a sudden change in habits should not harm the body.

natural urges

Natural Urges for	Consequences and pathological symptoms of suppression of urges	Possible Therapies
URINE	Pain in bladder, urinary region and passage, difficulty in passing urine, headache, distended lower abdomen	Tub bath, massage, fomentation, enema, urethral and vaginal douche.
FECES	Colic pain, retained stool and flatus (gas), cramps in calf muscles, distensions of stomach	Enema, massage, tub bath, and laxative drinks.
SEMINAL DISCHARGE	Pain in genitals, general body aches, pain in cardiac region, obstructed urine.	Massage, tub bath, chicken soup, wine, non-greasy enema, milk, rice, sexual intercourse.
FLATUS (gas)	Retained wind, urine, feces, pain and exhaustion, abdominal diseases due to vata vitiation.	Oil massage, intake of unctuous foods and drinks, enema
VOMITING	Skin itching, black pigmentation on face, nausea, fever, and anaemia.	Induction of vomiting, fasting, non-greasy foods, physical exercise, purgation.
SNEEZING	Stiff neck, headache, facial paralysis, weakness of the sense organ	Massage and fomentation of head and neck regions, nasal drops, clarified butter (ghee) and other vata pacifying diet.

Natural Urges for	Consequences and pathological symptoms of suppression of urges	Possible Therapies
ERUCTATION (belching)	Hiccups, anorexia, tremors, feeling of obstruction in cardiac region	Chest and back massage, take crystal sugar (*misri*)
YAWNING	Convulsions, numbness, tremor and shaking of the body	Food and other measures to pacify *vata*
HUNGER	Weakness, poor complexion, malaise, loss of appetite, giddiness.	Light, warm and unctuous food
THIRST	Dryness of throat and mouth, deafness, exhaustion, weakness, cardiac pain.	Sweet cold drinks
TEARS	Eye diseases, heart diseases, loss of appetite, giddiness	Wine, good sleep and consoling conversation
SLEEP	Drowsiness, headache, heaviness in eyes, malaise	Massage of the body and sound sleep
BREATHING	Heart diseases, fainting, tumours	Rest and *vata* pacifying measures

Nurturing the body

According to Ayurveda, taking food is like performing a *yajna* (fire sacrifice), only in this ritual we give obeisance to the digestive fire instead of a sacrificial fire. If you partake of a wholesome diet, you will enjoy the blissfulness of a healthy life.

Breakfast

Breakfast should be light in summer when the gastric fire is slow; it should be substantial when the fire is strong and when the weather is cold. The gastric fire slowly gains strength as the day advances; hence, the morning is not a conducive time to digest heavy and large meals. At the same time not eating at all also dampens the digestive fire, so beginning the day without giving fuel to the fire (*agni*) is like starting for a long drive without any fuel in your vehicle. Fasting is not reccommended at the beginning of the day.

Depending upon the season and the individual constitution, one can start the day with nutritionally sound food. You can choose to have fresh and nourishing fluids in the form of vegetable juice, for example: carrots, beetroot, cucumber and a little ginger (not meant for diabetics) or fruit juices (apple, pear, grape). Orange juice, however, is contraindicated on an empty stomach, as it is too acidic. Eat sweet and juicy fruits, followed by cereals depending upon the time of the year. Since food choices presented to us are so enormous, giving specific advice in this regard loses its significance.

To make milk easy for digestion, it should be boiled with a pinch of nutmeg for mover (vata), cardamom for transformer (pitta) and a slice of fresh ginger for binder (kapha)

Following the general rules of Ayurvedic dietetics, one can say that if a lean mover (*vata*) person has to have porridge, he or she needs to have wheat porridge, cooked in milk and sugar with nuts and a dash of cinnamon and eaten while it is hot. A transformer (*pitta*) person can have the same warm porridge but without nuts. But if a binder (*kapha*) person has to have porridge, it should be hot barley porridge cooked with vegetables, rock salt and ginger.

To make milk easy for digestion, it should be boiled with a pinch of nutmeg for mover (*vata*), cardamom for transformer (*pitta*) and a slice of fresh ginger for binder (*kapha*).

Other choices for breakfast are whole wheat bread with raw honey, stewed apple or pear with cloves added to it, raisins and figs soaked overnight, soaked almonds minus the skin with warm milk, mangoes followed by milk, sweetened *amlaki* (Indian gooseberry), or whole wheat bread stuffed with raw or cooked vegetables, with

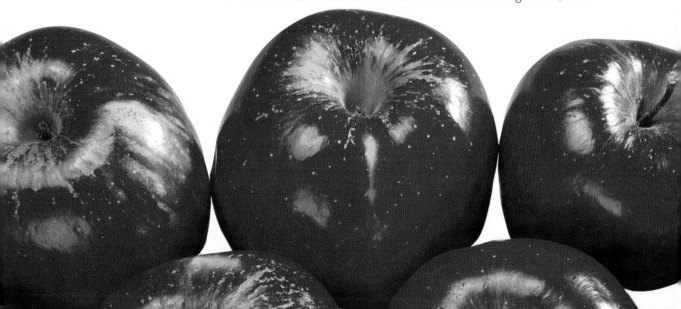

a little clarified butter. One can also blend together nuts, spices, fruit and milk, and have it warm or cool. One of these energy drinks includes a preparation of almonds crushed with a pinch of cinnamon and blended with warm milk. The idea is to have a fresh, nourishing meal that imparts strength but keeps the body light.

By focussing on basic functions of the human body like digestion, circulation and elimination, Ayurveda encourages the individual to make the right choices according to the bodily capacity. This goes a long way in correcting the life style mistakes and restoring the balance of the body.

At Work

One of the best things you can do, without disrupting regular work, is to simply breathe deeper for your health. Most of the time, we are engaged in shallow breathing, without realizing that it is resulting in blocked respiratory channels and fatigue. When you breathe deeply, the oxygen that reaches the brain makes it function better, purifies the blood and lifts the energy level of the body. One has to be observant of the quality of the air one breathes at home or at the work place. Keep air-purifying plants like basil (*tulsi*) and neem (*Azadirachta indica*) indoors and also keep checking the moisture level indoors.

Lunch: The main meal of the day

Lunch should be the main and the largest meal of the day. The sun is strongest at noon; correspondingly, transformer (*pitta*); the heat element, is strongest in our body, between 12 noon to 2 pm. The digestive fire is strong and the body is able to digest a wide variety of foods.

Ideally one should have all the six flavours (*rasas*) in one's meals. Lunch should be freshly cooked and warm. Cold meals depress the digestive fires. The same thing can be said about fast foods, frozen or canned food, and leftovers from the previous day or foods having preservatives or additives. They are low in

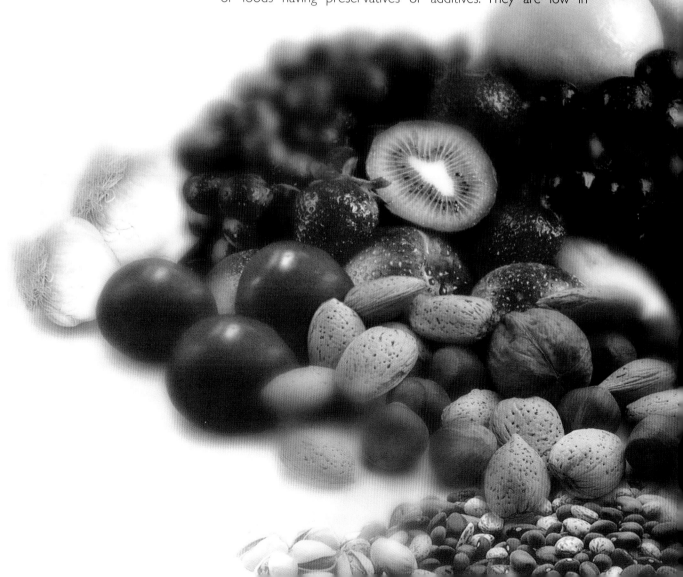

nutrition and heavy on digestion. If one is faced with a low energy level, body aches or stomach disorders, the first place to look for the cause is in one's diet. It is possible that one has adapted energy depleting foods in one's daily food regimen. It is best to have a closer look at what one is eating, break the old eating pattern if required and feast on the bounty which nature has provided us with abundance.

Since lunch should be the main meal, one needs to plan it in such a way as to make it nutritionally sound and fulfilling.

Ideally a meal that includes grains, beans or lentils, vegetables, spices and a yogurt drink (*lassi*) or buttermilk helps in digesting the food is wholesome, nutritious and balanced. One need not stick to rice and wheat as main grains, other grains such as millet, barley, buckwheat, quinoa, and couscous can be included alternatively on other days. Accordingly, lunch should consist of some vegetables, some grains, and some higher-protein foods like legumes, lentils, chickpeas, soya or milk cottage cheese. Non-vegetarian food like chicken or fish or any other meat should be eaten at lunchtime only.

Ayurveda is also particular about rules of consuming water with meals. One should have only a small amount of water along with meals, and more water only after a gap from the meal. However, the water should be either warm or of normal temperature but never cold. Cold water hinders the processes of digestion, metabolism and assimilation.

Lunch, should be eaten sitting down, in a comfortable position accompanied by compatible people and in pleasant surroundings.

The general rule for **mover (*vata*)** dominant people is to have warm food and sweet preparations. Caffeine has a dehydrating effect hence it disturbs the mover (*vata*), so one can have hearbal tea. During lunch, avoid cold salads, cold drinks, iced drinks, frozen desserts and hot spices; instead, have warm, unctuous food like grains, nuts and seeds. Vegetables need to be cooked as well. Only small amounts of greens can be had as salads. Wholewheat products (bread, tortillas), steamed rice, and oatmeal cooked in lot of water are healthy. Buttermilk made from fresh yoghurt (one part yogurt and six part water with roasted cumin seeds powder and salt) should become part of the meal.

Transformer (*pitta*) dominant people should have juicy, cooling foods with high water content. Avoid hot spicy foods (with chilies, peppers, etc.), avoid fried foods, vinegar, yogurt and cheese (take instead homemade cheese, and cottage cheese). The main meal should consist of wheat products, white basmati rice or barley or oats or amaranth. Legumes should be mung beans or small kidney beans; all others should strictly be in moderation. Juicy seasonal vegetables are allowed, but avoid spinach and tomatoes. Sweet buttermilk is also allowed, if they so desire.

Binder (*kapha*) people should eat mainly cooked vegetable and legumes, with a proportionately smaller helping of grains spiced according to taste (salt should be taken sparingly). They should avoid sweet desserts, cheese and meat. Reduce wheat and rice and replace with barley, millet, corn, buckwheat, rye, quinoa and oats. All vegetables and green, leafy vegetables (avoid sweet potatoes and tapioca) are advised. Take salted butter-milk with cumin, a pinch of dry ginger powder and black pepper powder.

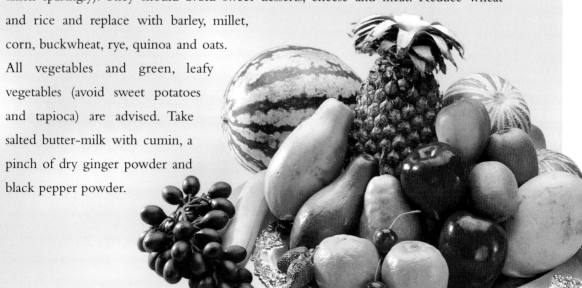

If one does not feel hungry at mealtimes, or if one feels heavy and sluggish in an hour or two after a meal, these indicate that the digestive fire is weak and needs to be treated by digestion enhancers. One such remedy is to eat a piece of fresh ginger with little lemon juice and rock salt before a full meal. It kickstarts the digestive juices and aids digestion. Alternatively, chew roasted fennel seeds (*saunf*) after the meal; this helps with digestion and keeps the breath fresh.

Instead of caffeine which adds to the stress level, when hunger or thirst strikes again, one can have lemon tea, ginger tea or plain warm water which helps in detoxifying the body. If one is feeling hungry later in the day, eat healthy snacks like raisins, dates, almonds, walnuts, salted or plain puffed rice and juicy fruits. It helps to change the eating pattern according to change in seasons. For instance, one can enjoy roasted sesame seeds (*til*) or roasted groundnuts and other delicacies made out of them in winters; they are warming and provide nourishment. The basic principle behind dietary choice is to eat according to the requirement of one's own body so as to ensure maximum health. The idea is to enhance the body's own internal awareness of itself and evolve a strategy of living which minimizes the risk of ill health. Oversights can be easily remedied if one works in that direction. It is certain that our bodies are already dealing with food related stresses. It may be necessary to change your eating patterns and incorporate and adapt to those foods which are essential to your specific constitution. The golden rule is to create balance wherever it is lacking.

Evenings

Evenings are the times when two phases of the sun meet. Nature is at rest, if one observes carefully, nature's rhythms are reflected in our bodily rhythms. Evenings offer a bodily calmness for offering prayers and sitting in meditation. It is a process of self-healing of the body-mind continuum.

Dinner

During the night, the digestive powers are not strong enough to digest a large quantity of food and heavy food preparations. One should avoid a large dinner. The later we eat, the less quantity should be consumed Usually dinner should consist of light, easy to digest foods. It is best to avoid heavy foods like yogurt, dense desserts, meats and cold food. These can lie dormant in the stomach and remain undigested for many hours.

Ayurveda recommends strolling after the evening meal (minimum 100 steps). Relaxing activities rather than strenuous activities (physical or mental) in the evening are more conducive to a restful sleep.

Bedtime

The rest cycle starts at night. During this rest period, the body withdraws from outside activities and gathers itself to regenerate and recuperate for the next day's activities. The body has an innate ability to heal and correct its imbalances; one has to only ensure that the rest cycle is not tempered with.

Although Ayurveda considers sexual activity an essential part of one's day-to-day activities, reckless indulgence is advised against. With a marked emphasis on foreplay, Ayurveda advises to abstain from sexual activity without having food or after consuming excess food; with a woman who is menstruating, with a woman/man or who does not have passionate desire for the other; if married to somebody else, or after strenuous exercise and in a place offering no privacy for such an act.

With the sole exception of summer and the monsoon season (too much indulgence in sex during these seasons vitiates the bodily vitalities) all other seasons are deemed fit to enjoy sexual activity.

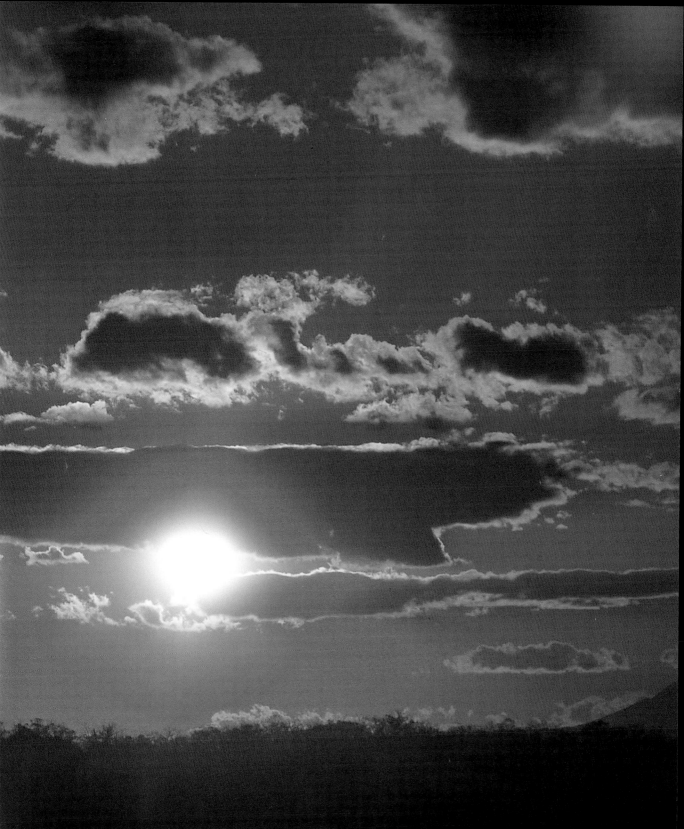

Weekly Cycle

~

Enema ~ Body Care

The weekly cycle refers to civic holidays after a week of work. Roughly one fortnight matches well with the natural unit tied to one phase of the lunar cycle.

Enema

As a purification measure, an enema is one of the most effective therapeutic tools to keep the *doshas* in balance. It alleviates *vata,* pacifies *pitta* and expels *kapha* which has got stuck in the colon.

Enemas are given according to one's constitution, age, season, and aggravated *doshas* or as a simple internal cleanser at any given point of time. If required, it should become part of the weekly routine.

Though people do take enemas without any help, it is advisable to first learn from a qualified physician and then start practicing alone. Enemas not only prevent diseases from taking root in the body, they also act as a therapy for old or new maladies which can make the body dysfunctional, like joint pains, gastrointestinal disorders and many other diseases due to vitiated *doshas*.

As a cleansing therapy, an enema is compared to the way in which the sun works. According to Ayurveda, just as the sun can take away the moistures from the earth to the sky, similarly, an enema captures the impurities from the soles of the feet to the head, even though it is done through the colon. Applied properly, there is no other therapy which can equal its efficacy in balancing disorders of the body.

Body Care

Earlier we talked about various cleansing routines during the daily regimen. Preoccupations of various kinds (work, home) can leave little time for an elaborate massage every day. Fix a day when you can take time out for full body massage, head massage, enema and a therapeutic bath.

Head Massage

Massaging the head has been given a very important place in Ayurveda. When a child is born, the top of the child's head (fontanel) is covered immediately with cloth soaked in oil (*bala taila*). This is to strengthen the head, sight and intelligence.

The head massage nourishes and strengthens all the body openings – especially the nose, eyes, ears, mouth and the top of the head. According to Indian tradition the soul goes out from here at the time of death. It is also the seventh wheel (*cakra*) of the human body.

During a head massage, certain vital points (*marmas*) on the head get a pressure treatment, resulting in enhanced immunity, treatment of the pituitary and the pineal glands, a strong nervous system and improved alertness of the body.

It keeps the *vata* in balance (some of the diseases that affect the brain like Parkinson's, Alzheimer's, some types of mental illnesses, are being recognized as diseases striking a 'dry brain' a *vatic* quality).

It does not let *kapha* accumulate in the head. People with a cold or sinusitis should have a head massage with warm oil and wrap the head with a scarf or a cap and not expose themselves to cold air after the massage.

A head massage keeps the *pitta* pacified. It is also beneficial in alleviating nose bleeds, burning eyes, and headaches.

First, put some oil on the top of the head, the first vital point (the *adhipati marma*), the crown, and start rubbing it in gently through fingers, massage this point gently for some time. Then oil all the roots on the scalp and massage the entire scalp area, going back and forth and to the sides of the head.

The second vital point is in the middle end of the scalp. It is also the place where we see hair forming a whirl. If we part our hair on the top of the head, this point (called *sikha*) is right at the end of hair parting. Pour some more oil on this point and massage with care.

The third vital point is where the skull meets the neck, massage the entire hair line near the neck with little pressure to improve circulation and cure stiff neck, it relieves headaches and takes away fatigue due to mental strain.

Finally, the ear lobes and the area surrounding the ears, specially the *utsepa marma*, the temporal bone.

If you have a weak body frame or have a high or low blood pressure then this would be the end of the head massage.

Otherwise, you can take the next step of the head massage and have a vigorous massage done on the head. In this, the palms as well as the fingers are used to give a rhythmic massage on the head. Both sides of the head are massaged with synchronized movements. It should be done with speed and pressure. After this vigorous massage, gently rub the head and tug the hair. This practice makes the roots stronger.

Wash your hair only after two hours.

Body Massage

Ayurvedic massage therapy becomes effective and more meaningful if one has a basic knowledge of (a) bodily type (b) choice of oils (c) vital points of the body (d) whether the massage needs to be a gentle or a stimulating one and (e) under what conditions massage is *not* to be given.

Once the bodily constitution is determined, start with the head then move from the neck, face, shoulders and chest to arms, then to midriff, and legs and finally to feet. Similarly while lying on the stomach, the upper back, the spinal column, the lower back and the back of the legs.

Hands and Arms: Give a long massage on the arms from shoulders towards the palms, and back again. Give a circular massage over the joints. Press the points on the arms with thumbs in circular motion. Press the hollow of the elbow and apply gentle pressure into the armpits.

Rub the oil on the hands; give a pressure massage to each finger. Massage the palms using both the thumbs, holding the back of the hands with the fingers. Massage the back of the hands. Give a pressure massage on each mound under all the fingers, giving more time to the spaces between the thumb and forefinger.

Hold the wrist firmly with the thumb and the fingers and give a pressure massage in circular motion.

A thorough massage of the arms and hands raises the immunity and strengthens all the organs of the body. It improves circulation and energizes the bodily tissues.

Chest, navel, abdomen: Give a gentle circular massage starting from the last rib from each side and move inwards and upward. Then, with both hands on the chest, use circular movements going towards the sides, navel and abdomen.

Indian tradition holds the navel to be the locus of the entire body. It is the place where all the circulatory channels are connected. Abdominal massage circulates

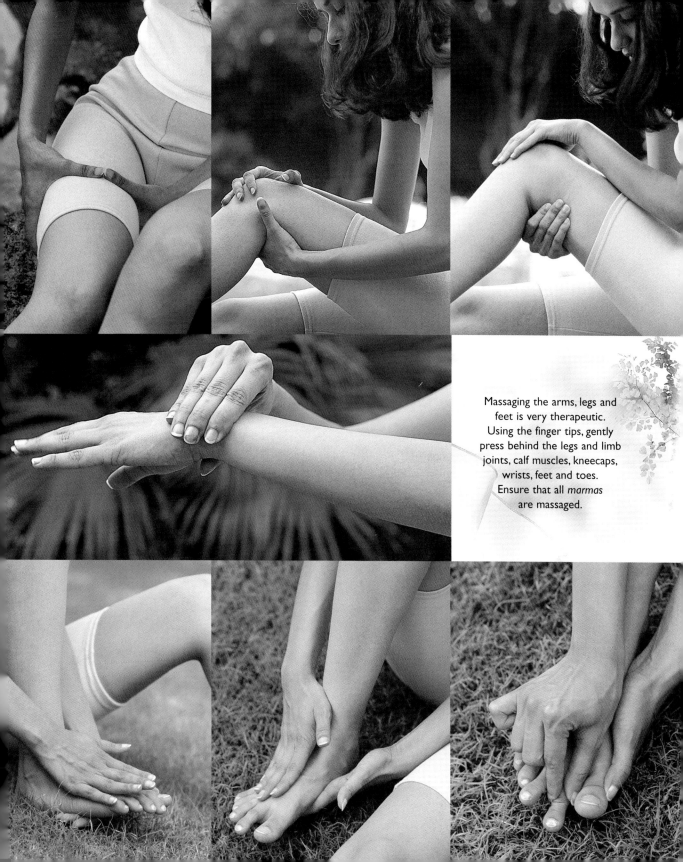

Massaging the arms, legs and feet is very therapeutic. Using the finger tips, gently press behind the legs and limb joints, calf muscles, kneecaps, wrists, feet and toes. Ensure that all *marmas* are massaged.

the energy in the navel region evoking strength and stability for the body.

Pour some oil in the navel; gently massage around the navel. Follow the colon from the right lower part of the abdomen, and move towards the left lower part of the abdomen. Do not apply any pressure on abdomen, navel or areas around navel.

Women are to be rubbed gently around the breasts. No pressure on the breasts or nipples is to be applied while massaging.

A chest and abdomen/navel massages improves the circulation, tones up the muscles, balances the *vata* in the abdomen and *kapha* in the chest.

Feet and Legs: Massaging the feet and legs is very therapeutic It provides total relaxation to the entire body. It is good for inducing sleep (treating insomniac conditions), removing dryness, improving circulation, reducing fatigue and numbness of the feet and increasing immunity of the body.

Rub the oil on the entire foot first. Hold the foot, use hands, palms and fingers to rub and massage thoroughly.

Give more time to the big toe, press the toe with the thumb and fingers several times, and rub with pressure the space between the big toe and the next finger under the foot.

Use the finger and thumb to massage each toe in circular motion and straight motion. Apply pressure on the tips of each toe and gently but firmly tug at them, one by one.

Give a vigorous massage on the soles of the feet, heels, joints, ankles and on both sides of the feet.

For the leg massage, use both hands to massage from knee towards ankles, giving special attention to calf muscles, kneecap and behind the knee joint, and the vital points on the outer and inner sides of the leg.

In the upper leg massage, start from the thigh joint moving towards the knee. A pressure massage can be given on the front and back of the upper leg.

Back Massage: Make the person lie on the stomach, resting the head and neck comfortably either on folded arms or soft cushions. For the back massage, the body should be in a relaxed posture, with its contours well placed. Oil the back and then start from the base of the vertebral column; make some circular movements with both the hands. Then place both your thumbs on both sides of the spinal column and start massaging towards the neck in small circular movements. Repeat this five or six times. Massage the upper back with open hands, especially all the vital points on the upper back, shoulder blades and around the buttocks.

The person can come back to the earlier position of lying on the back. Once again, some feather strokes can be applied on the entire body. The person should rest for a while before getting up. *Ubtana* and bathing should be only after two hours of full body massage.

When the body undergoes an oil massage, it experiences a feeling of warmth and nurturing. The Sanskrit word *'sneha'* stands both for oil and for love; oileation (*snehan*) undoubtedly heals the body (at the most subtle level) with love and care providing beauty, strength and stability to the bodily frame.

A typical *vata* skin is dry, cool and thin.
It has very fine pores and is delicate.

Skin Care

Ayurveda takes an integrated approach to skin care and beauty. Skin health or disorders are only part of the larger bodily wisdom. Skin responds and reacts in accordance with the choice of food, digestion and metabolism. The body's disposition to accumulate or expel waste reflects on the health of the skin since the skin also acts as an excretory organ that eliminates waste in the form of sweat.

How best one can assess the *dosha* imbalances goes a long way in restoring the health and natural beauty of the mind-body continuum.

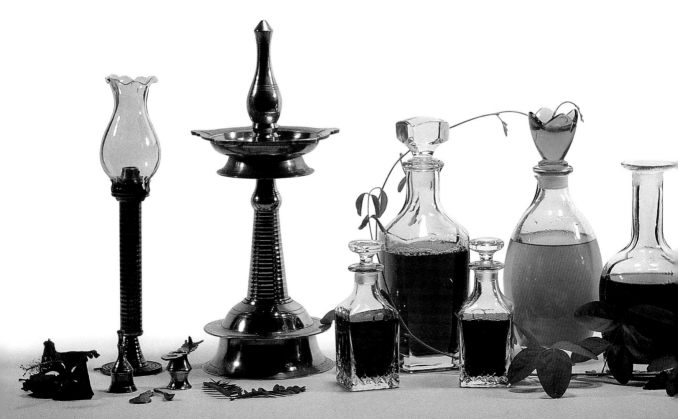

> Due to the element of fire in
> pitta people, the skin has a tendency
> towards being fair and has a glow

A typical *vata* skin is dry, cool and thin. It has very fine pores and is delicate. When the body has *vata* imbalance; the skin reflects this imbalance with a tendency to being rough, dry and coarse. It looks dull and sallow and is prone to early wrinkles. It can become predisposed towards dry eczema, flaky layers and various other skin ruptures. Mental stress flares up vatic skin conditions. Lack of sleep and intake of dry and rough foods can aggravate any skin problems.

Vata skin care involves re-hydrating the skin, since it has very little moisture of its own. If possible, this body type requires an oil massage every day. It also needs lubricating foods like *ghee* or clarified butter, sweet juicy fruits and other *vata* balancing foods in the diet. Taking care of worries, avoiding constipation and sleeping well are some of the preventive measures in vatic skin care regimen.

Due to the element of fire in *pitta* people, the skin has a tendency towards being fair and has a glow. It is warm and is neither translucent nor thick. *Pitta,* out of balance, makes this skin prone to acne, freckles, pigmentation, rashes and boils. *Pitta* skin is sensitive to heat and sunlight and can flare up under such conditions like excessive exercise and competitive sports. Emotions like anger, grief and stress add to the problems of the *pitta* skin types.

Pitta skin care involves avoiding excessive exposure to sunlight, drinking enough pure water, avoiding excessively spicy and salty

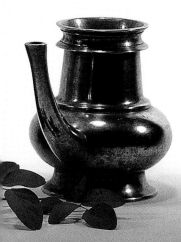

Kapha skin type is soft, and
relatively oily. It is sufficiently
moist, hence develops
wrinkles only at a later
stage in life.

foods. Intake of juicy fruits and other *pitta* balancing foods are to be incorporated in daily diet along with working towards emotional balance through calming yoga and breathing exercises.

Kapha skin type is soft, and relatively oily. It is sufficiently moist, hence develops wrinkles only at a later stage in life. *Kapha* imbalance makes this skin prone to clogged pores, wet eruptions, pimples and fungal infections of various kinds.

It is best to avoid oily foods and sweets. Herbs like ginger, garlic, *kapha* balancing foods and spices need to be added to daily diet. Moderate use of honey, purgative measures and vigorous exercise helps to correct the *kapha* imbalance. A dry friction massage, hot water and steam baths help to unclog the skin pores.

Dual *prakriti* skins like *vata-pitta*, *kapha-pitta* and *vata-kapha* manifest combined traits of the doshas. A judicious way to keep the balance is for *vata-pitta* skin is to follow a regimen of the *pitta* in summer and that of *vata* in winter. *Kapha-pitta* can follow a *kapha* skin regimen in winter and *pitta* skin regimen in summer.

Yearly Regimen

~

Pancakarma is a highly effective preventive and curative therapeutic tool in Ayurveda. Over time, we keep accumulating toxins from our food, our living spaces, our thoughts and above all, through a life style which tends to waver between healthy and unhealthy in many ways. *Pancakarma* is a therapy which weeds out deep-rooted impurities, wastes or toxins from the body. It balances the functions of the three vitalities. It rejuvenates and facilitates the innate capacity of the body to heal itself again.

Pancakarma is done in three phases. First, the preparatory phase *(purva karma)* consists of (a) internal or external oileation *(snehan)* of the body and (b) perspiration *(svedan)* of the body. Making the body perspire constitutes expulsion of bodily wastes in the form of sweat. These procedures soften and liquefy the vitiated *doshas* and bring them to the alimentary canal. These *doshas* are removed later through an appropriate purification regimen.

The second phase consists of the main procedure *(pradhana karma)*.

Five main procedures (with their various techniques) of *pancakarma* are:

> *Vamana* (drugs are given to induce vomiting),
> *Virechana* (therapeutic purgation),
> *Basti* (medicated enemas are given),
> *Nasya* (medicine given through nose)
> *Rakta moksana* (blood letting)

Induced Vomiting *(Vamana)*

In this therapy, vomiting is induced through medicines. It helps in disorders of *kapha dosha*. By this procedure, vitiated *doshas* are eliminated through the upper gastro-intestinal track. It is used in treating conditions ranging from chest congestion and asthma, to imbalances like hyperacidity. It should be done under the care of an experienced Ayurvedic physician.

Therapeutic Purgation *(Virechana)*

Vitiated *doshas* are removed through the rectum. Herbs having laxative qualities are given to induce a controlled purgation. It also cleanses the small intestine, kidney, lungs, sweat glands, liver and the gall bladder. It is used for treating diseases like jaundice, fever, skin disorders, arthritis, digestive disorders, and epilepsy.

Medicated Enema *(Basti)*

Through the anus, urinary organs and genitals, various kinds of enemas like water, oils and milk (medicated and non medicated) are given with a special instrument made for this purpose. It removes aggravated *vata* through the lower gastro-intestinal tract. This therapy, removes the *doshas*, cleanses the body of *ama* and wastes, balances the functions of the *doshas*, provides nourishment to bodily tissues and raises immunity. It treats all kinds of arthritis, obesity and numerous other diseases. Other bodily sites for administering *basti* are eyes, lower back, head and the chest region.

Medicated decoctions are applied on these bodily parts for therapeutic purposes.

Nasal medication *(Nasya)*

This amounts to putting medicated oils, decoctions or powders into the nasal passage. It alleviates sinusitis, migraines, headaches, epilepsy, and many other imbalances of the head and neck region.

Blood Letting (*Rakta Moksana*)

Blood letting is a selective and localized treatment in which vitiated blood is taken out by putting leeches or by inserting surgical instruments. It is used to treat diseases like eczema, leucoderma, herpes and gout.

The third phase of *pancakarma* consists of post-procedures *(pascata karma)* of special diets and daily regimen, which has to be strictly adhered to so that the newly purified bodily tissues *(dhatus)* get strengthened by these measures.

Not everyone can undergo this therapy. Those who are too young, the elderly, pregnant women and those too frail are not fit for this therapy. Similarly, emesis is not done on people with weak hearts; purgation is not to be done on alcoholic, wounded, bleeding or people suffering from high fever. The enema is not given to hungry, thirsty or emotionally disturbed people and those who suffer from respiratory problems.

Caution: *Pancakarma* should be done under the care of an experienced Ayurvedic physician.

Seasonal Regimen

~

Early Winter ~ Late Winter ~
Spring ~ Summer ~ Rains ~ Autumn

The outside environment affects the inner working of our body in a significant way. Ayurveda provides us with a consistent and detailed theory and practice of seasonal regimen.

Seasons affect the individual constitution in an intimate way. Ayurveda teaches us how to best adapt to the changing seasons and maintain a healthy, body-specific lifestyle. Nature provides us with many patterns, which change according to the seasons. To comprehend the nexus between bodily functions and seasonal variations, one has to watch nature very closely and at the same time observe the subtle changes in one's body.

Ayurveda divides the year into six seasons *(ritu)*, each corresponding to two months (one *ritu)*, which roll from one to the other in a cyclic way. The constitution of a person and seasons are deeply connected. A person's health has a direct relation to the climate he/she lives in. The changes that occur during each season directly affect the person's health and general well being. Since each individual has a specific body type, adjustment to these seasonal changes also varies according to the specific requirement of the person specific nature.

A person's health has a direct
relation to the climate he/she lives in.

74

*The end of one phase and beginning
of the other phase has been given
immense importance for following
preventive regimen to stay healthy
for the coming season.*

The annual journey of the earth around the sun manifests itself in six seasons. They correspond to the two directions of the sun's movement – the northern solstice and the southern solstice. When the sun is in the northern solstice, Ayurveda calls it *adanakala* (acquisition time: the sun takes away moisture and cooling properties from earth), when the sun is in the southern solstice it is called *visargakala* (parting time; the earth gets back its moisture after the sun's spell is over and the moon becomes powerful).

During the northern solstice, the sun and winds are very powerful; they take away moisture (*adana*) from the earth, and strength from the people. Health remains at low ebb during this period. The southern solstice brings back the strength, as the moon is more powerful. The earth acquires back its moisture through cold winds and rains.

The northern phase begins in mid January. With each month, the sun and winds becomes hotter and more aggressive. Culmination of this period starts from mid June, when the sun starts its southward journey. It approximates between mid July to mid January when the sun starts becoming milder, as rains and clouds restrain it. The moon becomes more powerful, releasing moisture and coolness to the earth.

These naturally occurring seasonal aberrations in the body can be checked through the preventive methods of Ayurveda and one can enjoy a state of perfect health throughout the year

The end of one phase and beginning of the other phase has been given immense importance for following preventive measures to stay healthy for the coming season.

The end of the southerly phase and the ushering in of the northerly phase and vice versa are considered important transitional phases. During the northerly phase, the aggressive sun and the harsh winds take away moisture from the atmosphere resulting in an enhanced state of pungent, astringent and bitter tastes in the substances. These three tastes have an emaciating effect on the body as such; they deplete the bodily tissues making it weak and prone to diseases.

During the southerly phase, when the earth and its creatures start regaining their moisture, sour, salty and sweet tastes become predominant, cooling, nourishing and strengthening the body when used in food substances.

These naturally occurring seasonal aberrations in the body can be checked through the preventive methods of Ayurveda and one can enjoy a state of perfect health through out the year.

This table is only an indication of the dominant tastes and dominant elements during the seasons. Neither the tastes nor the elements are ever mutually exclusive. Understanding the subtle relations among seasons, elements, tastes and the vitalities (*doshas*) is a big leap towards mastering the Ayurvedic way of living.

seasons, tastes and elements

Ritu	Seasons	Dominant Taste	Dominant Elements
Sisira	Late Winter	Tikta (hot and bitter)	Air & Space (akasa)
Vasanta	Spring	Kasaya (astringent)	Air & Earth
Grisma	Summer	Kattu (pungent)	Air & Fire
.Varsa	Rainy	Amala (sour)	Earth &Fire
Sarata	Autumn	Lavana (salty)	Water &Fire
Hemanta	Early Winter	Madhura (sweet)	Water & Earth

Six Seasons

~

Early Winter

The sun is mild, the moon becomes stronger and the winds are cold and dry. It is last season of the southerly phase of the sun. From the health point of view it is considered the best season. The digestive power is strong; it kindles inside the body and is capable of consuming any substance irrespective of its heaviness or its quantity. If this fire (*agni*) does not get its fuel, it affects the body tissues and the nutritive fluids, resulting in imbalance of the mover (*vata dosha*). Hence consuming less than required is

> As a routine, oil massage, exercise, smearing of turmeric paste (as *ubtana*) on body and a warm water bath are conducive to the body.

contraindicated. During winter, one should avoid food and drinks having pungent, bitter and astringent tastes, as they are cold and dry and will lead to vitiation of mover (*vata*) qualities. Sweet, sour and salty foods should dominate in the diet. In various food preparations it is advisable to use fresh ginger, dry ginger powder, rock salt, small cardamom, and coriander seed powder.

As a routine, oil massage, exercise, smearing of turmeric paste (as *ubtana*) on body and a warm water bath are conducive to the body. Protection from the cold, basking in the sun, long sleeping hours (nights being long) and a good amount of sexual activity keeps the mover (*vata*) in balance in this season.

Late Winter

Most of the regimen of early winter holds good for late winter as well; only as the months progress, the sun is gaining strength gradually, as its northward journey begins, the winds are becoming dry. Now the dominant tastes in food are bitter, pungent and astringent. Together they create a drying effect on the body and can create an imbalance in the mover (*vata*). A warm and nourishing diet high on salt, sour and sweet tastes, a warm dwelling place, warm clothing, oileation of the body and reduced sexual activities are all important to keep mover (*vata*) in balance. *Kapha prakriti* people need to be careful in this season so as not to vitiate *kapha*, as early winter food and drinks have been sweet, heavy and unctuous.

Spring

The sun is warm and gradually gains in strength and the winds are hot. *Kapha dosha* accumulated in winters (due to eating heavy, sweet and unctuous substances) is stimulated in this season. The heat of the sun liquefies the *kapha* and brings it to the fore. The result is a slowing down of the digestive fire and the body becomes susceptible to many binder-oriented (*kaphaj*) diseases and discomforts, like feelings of fatigue, colds and cough, congested lungs and so on.

Spring is a major seasonal transition. The body is vulnerable to diseases. However, spring is also a season for bodily cleansing. Before the binder (*kapha*) takes a root in the bodily tissues, elimination therapies like emesis, purgation and *sirovirecana* (elimination of doshas from the head) are good alternatives.

An early morning walk is highly recommended. A massage with sesame oil or applying sandalwood paste generally keeps the body in balance. Excretory orifices need to be cleaned with warm water.

Massage, gargling and care of the eyes should become part of one's daily routine. Sexual activity and exercise minimize the effect of *kapha* at this time. Sleeping during the day should be avoided.

> Food at this time of the year
> should have more of bitter,
> astringent and pungent
> tastes to pacify *kapha*

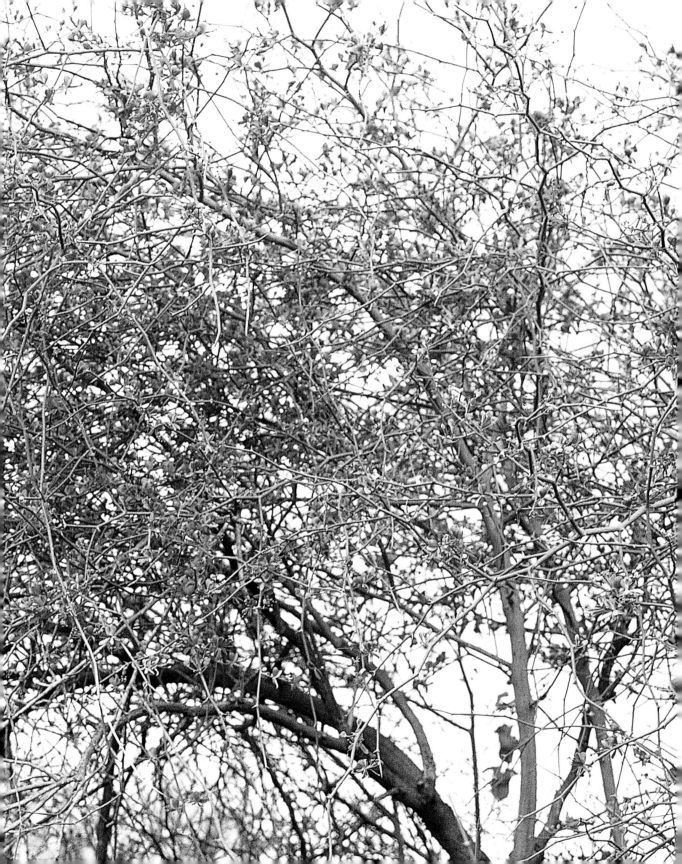

Food at this time of the year should have more of bitter, astringent and pungent tastes to pacify *kapha*. One needs to avoid taking heavy, unctuous, sour, fried, spicy and sweet diets on a regular basis. Barley and wheat are preferred grains during spring. Green gram (*mung*), red lentil (*masur*) and green vegetables should become part of everyday diet. Wood apple, pumpkin, bitter gourd, eggplant, fenugreek, small tender radish; garlic and lemon (to name a few) are considered wholesome in this season.

As a preventive regimen, one can take *haritaki* (*Terminalia chebula*, Indian gallut) powder with honey every day. It guards against colds and coughs, fever, indigestion and premature aging. It is not to be taken during pregnancy.

Summer

During this season, the severity of the sun reduces the element of water *(kapha)* in the body. Since there is an enhanced action of fire and air elements, *kapha* gets depleted, a bitter taste predominates and the body becomes rough and weak. Due to enhanced roughness and dryness, *vata* gets accumulated in the body (*vata* having the same qualities). But *vata* becomes erratic in the body, since *kapha* (on which the *vata* rides) is also reduced in the body. To balance the mover (*vata*) and binder *(kapha)* the body has to be nourished with sweet, cold and light food. Dehydration, diarrhea, sunstroke, vomiting, fainting, *pitta*-fevers, nosebleeds, and skin rashes are some of the avoidable maladies associated with imbalanced vitalities during the summer.

In summer, we need to take more cooling (not necessarily

cold) foods, like fresh, sweet seasonal fruits and juicy seasonal vegetables like gourds of various varieties, onions, cool salads like cucumber and lemon, but less of tomatoes. The diet should have light grains like boiled rice, and light pulses. Avoid yogurt and replace it with buttermilk. Food with pungent and salty tastes should be avoided. Cooling leaves of mint and coriander should be used in the regular diet as condiments (chutney, for example), as they keep the *vata* and pitta in balance and help digestion.

In summer, watermelon, melons, cucumber, pomegranate and mangoes make delicious snacking alternatives. Famous Indian *sharbats* (cooling drinks made from fruits and herbs i.e. raw mango, tamarind, lemon, mint etc.) are good for controlling excessive thirst, replacing the fluid loss due to heat, helping the digestion and providing nourishment to the body.

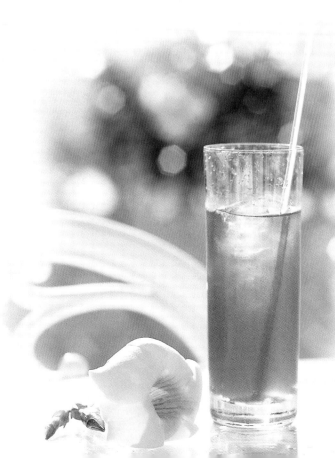

If possible, outdoor activities should be done in the morning and evening, avoiding going under the direct sun. Drinking cold water immediately after one has come from outside (hot weather) is harmful. Exercise, which leads to lot of sweating, is to be done sparingly, sexual activities need to be reduced. A short afternoon nap is rejuvenating.

One should enjoy the pleasures of the scent of flowers, cool water and gentle body rubs with cooling oils, such as sandalwood oil.

Rainy Season

With the rains the southerly phase of re-hydration begins. The body's powers, weakened through heat and dehydration during summer, is further weakened during the rainy season, or monsoon. The digestive power is already weak, and gets further weakened by an imbalance of *vata* and other vitalities *(doshas)*. Vapourization from the earth in this season affects *vatic* element in the body, the dampness in the atmosphere affects the body's digestive powers and metabolism. It is moist and humid outside the body, which enhances the same elements inside the body. *Agni* or fire is at its lowest and needs to be treated accordingly. The number of diseases that occur during the rainy season exceed all other seasons. Ayurveda mentions stomach disorders like indigestion, diarrhea, dysentery, many kinds of fevers, worms infestation, jaundice, breathing trouble, cough and colds, headaches, body aches and various skin diseases.

As a routine, undertake a dry friction massage of the body; keep the skin, skin folds, and spaces between the fingers and toes absolutely dry. Wear light clothes.

Since the digestive power is weak, one needs to have a light and nourishing diet with the predominance of salt and sour

> Since the digestive power is weak, one needs to have a light and nourishing diet with the predominance of salt and sour tastes. Wheat, seasonal vegetables and soups should be part of the diet

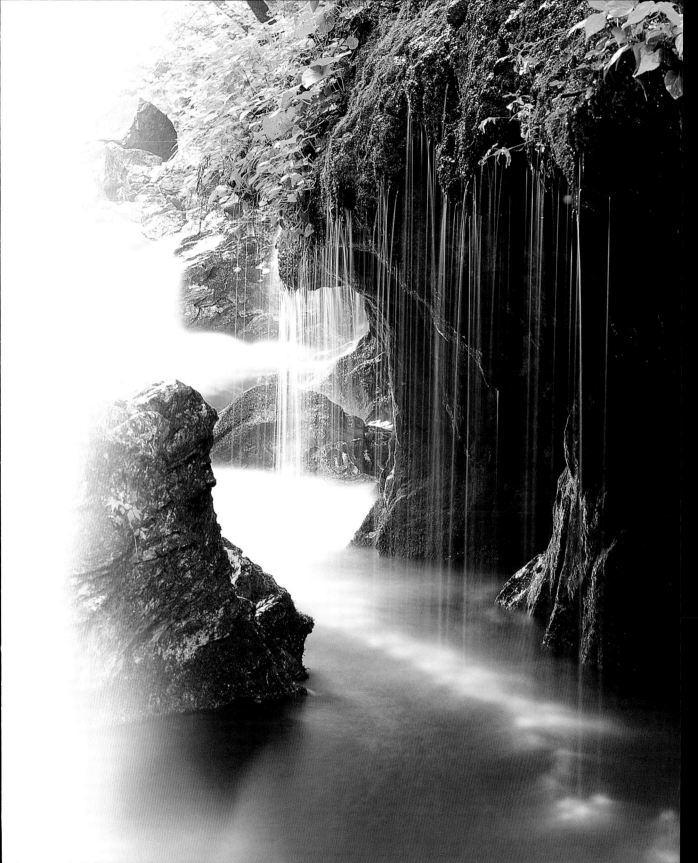

tastes. Wheat, seasonal vegetables and soups should be part of the diet.

Dry ginger powder and *heeng* (asafoetida) can be liberally used while cooking the food (not to be used in *pitta* aggravated situations); similarly, honey is best for keeping the inner bodily dampness in check.

One can include fresh soup of green gram, ginger, onions, garlic, cumin and fennel in the daily diet.

As a routine for the rainy season avoid napping during the day, as it vitiates *kapha.*

Avoid excessive exercise and excessive indulgence in sexual activities; it can vitiate *pitta.* Avoid moving about in the sun and live in a house devoid of humidity.

Purgation becomes necessary to expel *pitta* from the body. One can take any one of these substances at night like castor oil (a teaspoon in warm milk at bed time), psyllium husk (*isabgol,* two tablespoons in water at bed time), *triphala* (two tablespoons with water at bed time).

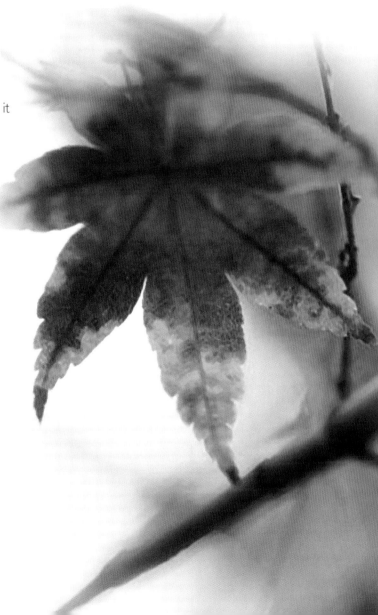

Autumn

Pitta, which accumulates during the rainy season, gets vitiated in autumn. The digestive powers, which are weakened in the rainy season do not become strong immediately. Since *pitta* increases in this season, conditions associated with this imbalance are hyperacidity, ulcers, stomach-aches, and other digestive disorders. When *pitta* gets vitiated, blood too tends to vitiate, and this gets manifested in many skin conditions like boils, eruptions burning in the eyes etc. One needs to avoid direct sunlight, sleeping in the afternoon and eating yourt.

One should eat only when hungry and not fill the stomach completely. Food should be chosen so as not to increase *pitta*.

Food and drinks, which are sweet, light, cold and bitter should be taken. Rice, barley, and wheat are the grains best consumed in this season.

One needs to avoid sesame, tamarind, sour and dry foods, mustard oil and wines.

Purgation is the only remedy to clear the body of excess *pitta*. Clarified butter made out of cow's milk is also a *pitta* pacifier. One can take a spoonful of *triphala* powder at night to clear the system. Other substances that can be used for purgation are raisins, liquorices and castor oil.

The moon in the season of *Sarada* is considered extremely beneficial for all living beings. Exposure to this moonlight nourishes the body. The famous *Sarada purnima* (full moon) festival in India celebrates this event.

Ritu Sandhi or the cusp of two Seasons

There are two major transitional phases of the sun falling in summer (southerly phase begins) and the early winter (when the northerly phase begins). And there are six major seasonal transitions. The last week of the previous season and the first week of the new season are called the cusp or *ritusandhi,* where two seasons meet. According to Ayurveda most of the vitality *(dosha)* imbalances occur at this time. The body becomes susceptible to diseases and disorders. We are advised to cross this period with care.

People do tend to fall sick at the change of seasons because the body carries over the accumulated toxins from the previous season, which become manifest at the advent of a new season. So a dietary adjustment and conscious measure to balance these vitalities *(doshas)* needs to be taken at the appropriate time. One can pass through these transition periods by changing some diet patterns, increasing or decreasing some of the tastes in one's foods and with some modification of the habits and lifestyle.

The faulting vitalities *(doshas)* exit the body through the orifices, i.e. the bowel, bladder, stomach, lungs (through the mouth) and pores of the skin. Ayurveda provides us with the herbs and diets, which can act as laxatives, diuretics, emetics (induce vomiting), and clear mucus from the body and also help the body to sweat *(svedana).*

Dosha	Season of accumulation	Season of aggression	Season of calm
mover (*vata*)	Summer	Rains Late winter	Autumn
transformer (*pitta*)	Rainy season	Autumn Rainy season	Early winter
binder (*kapha*)	Early winter	Spring Rainy season	Summer

Seasonal behaviour of the three *doshas*

The transition from one season to another is rarely an abrupt one. We prepare for the coming season by changing our diet, regimen and clothing. We take out umbrellas in anticipation of the coming rains and we are prepared with warm clothes before winter. Similarly, while one season is going to change into the other, it is imperative to follow a regimen that decreases that particular *dosha*, which is likely to get aggravated in the coming season. For instance, follow a *kapha* decreasing diet at the end of winter before it gets aggravated in spring – you will avoid coughs and colds and congested lungs. All that is required is to be synchronized with the inner and outer rhythms of the body.

Making an effort once will make all subsequent efforts come naturally.

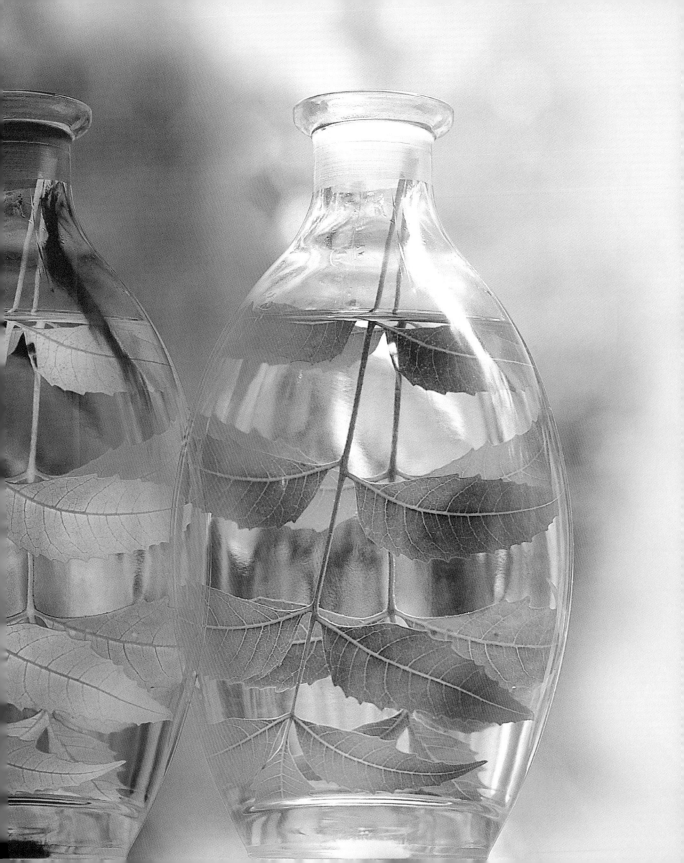

regulating the
ayurvedic way
~

Food Regimen and Incompatible Foods

According to the Vedantic classification of human embodiment, there are five sheaths (*koshas*) or envelopes that enclose the *atman* (self). The *anandamaya-kosha* closely corresponds to the spiritual soul or state of pure bliss; the second is the *vijnanamaya-kosha*, or thoughts and ideas (the higher *manas*); third, the *manomaya-kosa*, the will and the desires (lower *manas* with *kama*), making the human soul; fourth, the *pranamaya-kosha*, the vital-astral soul or *prana* and *linga-sarira* (subtle body); and lastly, the *annamaya-kosha*, the food body, the physical body or *sthula-sharira*.

A sensible consumption of food is responsible for health and longevity. Do not indulge in an unhealthy diet either out of greed or ignorance.

Ayurveda provides us with details of the sources and composition of food substances, their nutritive value, their action on the body and rules of consuming food. It is difficult to do justice to the entire science of food and nutrition as propounded by Ayurveda in these pages. We will, however, touch upon some of the basic aspects of Ayurvedic dietetics in this chapter.

The gross body (*sthula sarira*) as explained earlier, is composed of five elements. The sustenance and nourishment of the human body is dependent on his intake from the outer world. The five elements comprising the body and its intake are: *akasa* (space or ether), *vayu* (air), *tejas* (fire), *apa* (water) and *prithvi* (earth), which constitute the physical basis of the body, where as the three *doshas*, *vata*, *pitta* and *kapha* are the biological basis of the human body in terms of which the *prakriti*, or the individual constitution and *vikriti* (deviation from the constitution) can be explained and understood. When it comes to food and medicine, the composition and their properties are described through the five elements whereas their actions on the body are understood through three *doshas*. Again, the three *doshas* are found only in a living being whereas five elements are found in the entire living and nonliving realms.

Rasa is another concept that is quite central to the Ayurvedic theory of food and nutrition. *Rasa* in this context means 'taste' which is either an inherent property or an acquired property of a substance (*dravya*). *Rasa* also stands for the end product of digestion and it also stands for a particular *dhatu* of the body.

There are six tastes – *madhur* (sweet), *amla* (sour), *lavana* (salt), *katu* (pungent), *tikta* (bitter) and *kashaya* (astringent). Primarily, water is the substratum for the manifestation of different tastes.

After tasting a substance, one comes to know of its heating or cooling potentials (*virya*), and only after few hours or the next day one comes to know the post digestive effect of the substance consumed (*vipaka*) on the body.

It is important to know and understand the *rasas* along with the substances through which they act on the *doshas* because they increase or vitiate *doshas* and decrease or pacify *doshas*.

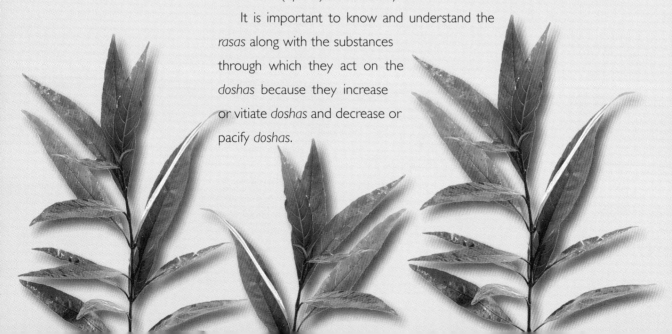

Sweet (*madhura*)

Sugar (in all forms), such as brown or white, raw, refined, molasses, sugar cane juice, honey and so on. Grains like wheat, rice, barley, and corn. Milk and milk products like *ghee* (clarified butter), butter, and cream. Most sweet fruits like mangoes, grapes, banana, dates, pears, melons, figs and dry fruits like almonds. Cooked vegetables like beetroot, carrot, potato, sweet potato, and cauliflower. This also includes oils like sesame oil, groundnut oil, corn oil, palm and sunflower oil (post digestive).

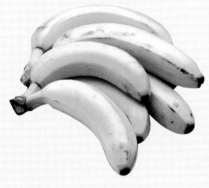

Sour (*amla*)

Includes products such as lemons, limes, oranges, pineapples, cherries, plums, Indian gooseberry (*amlaki*), tamarind, unripe mango, mango powder, pomegranate seeds and pickled vegetables. Sour milk products like yogurt, buttermilk, curds, cheese and sour cream etc. Most of the wines and carbonated beverages, vinegars, and soy sauce are sour.

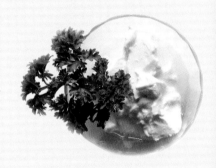

Salty (*lavana*)

Salts of all kinds: rock salt, sea salt, salt from the ground and foods to which salt has been added for example, pickles, nuts etc.

Pungent (*katu*)

Most of the spices, like chilies, black pepper, long pepper, cloves, mustard seeds, turmeric, ginger, dried ginger, cumin, cloves, garlic, etc. Also, raw vegetables like radish, onion.

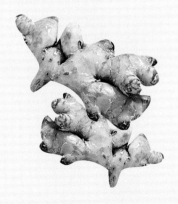

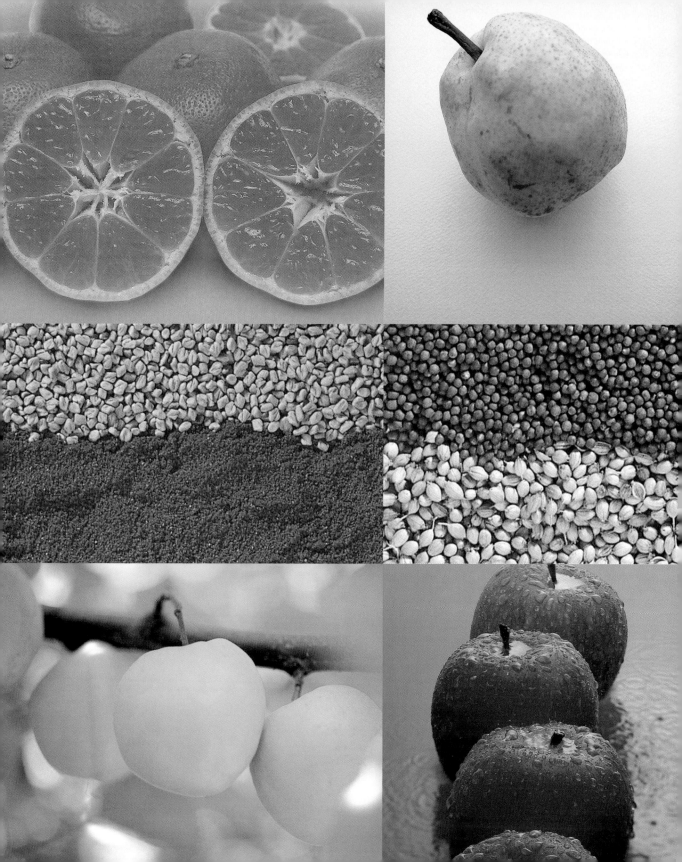

Bitter (*tikta*)

This includes *neem*, bitter gourd, sandalwood and marigold and fruits like olives. Leafy vegetables like spinach, green cabbage. Spices like fenugreek and turmeric.

Astringent (*kasaya*)

Astringent tastes include honey, walnuts, hazelnuts and cashews. Most of the pulses (legumes), i.e., beans, lentils, peas, beans; also, most raw vegetables and sprouts, lettuce, green leafy vegetables. Fruits like pomegranate, berries like blackberry and cranberry, and most unripe fruits.

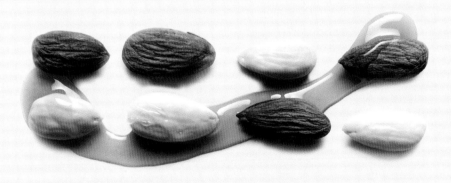

Actional Qualities of Material Substances

All substances are classified according to the qualities they possess. These are called *gunas*. *Gunas* are the pointers towards the material composition of a substance and an absolutely essential yardstick to know the nature of a substance. *Gunas* sometimes dominates the *rasas* and *vipaka*. For instance, water being sweet increases *kapha* (binder) but if it is hot it decreases *kapha* (binder).

Qualities like heavy, light, cold, hot, dry and unctuous are most commonly used by people in day-to-day life to qualify food substances. For instance, ginger is given to help cure colds and coughs. Sandalwood is given in summer to impart its coolness on the body.

The most important point is that it is the *guna* that provides the foundational ground for explaining both health and disease. *Gunas* act on the principle that similar qualities will increase the *dosha*, and dissimilar or opposite qualities will decrease the *dosha*. For instance, anything dry almost always increases *vata* (mover), which is brought to balance by unctuous substances like oils etc. Anything hot increases *pitta* (transformer). So the cooling substances pacify the *pitta* (transformer) and anything heavy can increase *kapha* (binder), to balance *kapha* (binder) those substances are required, which have light and dry qualities.

Modern medicine's new found interest in food and dietetics marks a paradigm shift in its perspective on health and disease. Food till recent years was regarded useful only for the upkeep of the bodily processes involving statistically measured proteins and carbohydrates for the growing human body. The relevance of food and the effective role it can play in the preventive and therapeutic domains is increasingly being recognized by contemporary biomedicine.

Ayurveda's approach to classify food substances is very different from the modern way of understanding various food groups i.e. grains, dairy, vegetables, fruits and meats. Ayurveda goes a step further. It provides us with a consistent approach for arriving at a more customized, balanced diet according to a person's individual constitution.

Based on the principles of Ayurveda, we have tried below to give a qualitative profile of some of the basic food groups. These tables are not exhaustive, since food substances are far too many and too diverse to be accommodated in these pages. We are providing only indicators to know the food substances, their qualities and their actions vis-à-vis bodily vitalities. Knowing one's constitution and then determining the nutritional requirement of the body can go a long way in preserving and maintaining good health for a life time.

Common name of the food	Qualities	Effects on Vitalities	Effects on various bodily processes
Rice	Light, sweet, cold, unctuous, stable	Increases slightly, *vata* and *kapha* pacifies *pitta*	Promotes strength
Wheat	Unctuous, heavy, cold, sweet, slightly astringent, purgative	Decreases *vata*, *pitta* increases *kapha*	Provides strength, helps broken bones to join faster, bulk promoting
Barley	Cold, sweet, heavy, dry, astringent, pungent after digestion	Increases *vata*, decreases *pitta*, *kapha*	Diuretic, alleviates thirst, ignites fires
Maize	Dry	Increases *vata*, decreases *pitta*, *kapha*	

New cereals are heavy, old crop is light

Common name of the food	Qualities	Effects on Vitalities	Effects on various bodily processes
Green Gram (*mung*)	Dry, light, sweet, astringent, cold, pungent after digestion	Slightly increases *vata*, *kapha* decreases *pitta*,	Strength giving, helps in wound healing, considered best pulse
Kidney beans (*rajma*)	Light, cold, sweet after digestion	Increases *vata*, decreases *pitta* , *kapha*	Causes heat in the body
Lentil (*masur*)	Light, cold, dry, sweet, sweet after digestion	Increases *vata*, decreases *pitta* , *kapha*	Strength giving
Sesame (*til*)	Heavy, unctuous, hot, pungent, astringent, bitter, pungent after digestion	Destroys *vata*, removes accumulated *pitta* and *kapha* in the abdomen	Good for skin, teeth. Increases breast milk, promotes strength.

Common name of the food	Qualities	Effects on Vitalities	Effects on various bodily processes
Millet *(jwar, bajra, raagi)*	Cold, dry, astringent, heavy on digestion	Decreases *pitta* and *kapha*	May cause constipation
Pumpkin	Heavy, cold, alkaline	Pacifies *vata, kapha*	Strengthens *agni*, causes constipation,
Water melon	Heavy, unctuous, cold	Pacifies *vata, pitta* Increases *kapha*	Nourishing, diuretic, refreshing
Melon	Cold, heavy	Alleviates *pitta*	Nourishing, decreases semen
Eggplant	Hot, sweet, light, pungent after digestion	Decreases *vata*, increases *pitta*, decreases *kapha*	Blood forming, diuretic, strengthens *agni*, induces sleep
Cucumber	Cold, dry, heavy, sweet, sour	Alleviates *pitta, kapha*	Diuretic, helps in difficulty in passing urine
Bitter gourd	Light, bitter, cold	Increases *vata*, decreases, *pitta, kapha*	Helps in breaking fecal matter from the intestines
Yam	Light, pungent, pungent after digestion	Increases *vata, kapha*	Causes constipation, used in breathing disorders

Old crop of pulses is rough and light, the new is heavy.
Pulses are digested easily when cooked with spices and a little ghee.

Common name of the food	Qualities	Effects on Vitalities	Effects on various bodily processes
Potato	Dry, sweet, heavy, cold, sweet after digestion	Increases *vata, kapha*	Causes constipation, hard to digest, gives strength
Radish (tender)	Light, hot	Increases *pitta, kapha*	Kindles digestive fire, given in jaundice
Radish (ripe)	Dry, hot	Vitiates *vata, pitta, kapha*	
Carrot	Sweet, bitter, hot, light,	Decreases *vata, kapha*	Given for the treatment of intestinal worms
Garlic	Unctuous, hot, heavy, pungent, sweet, pungent after digestion	Decreases *vata, kapha*	Used in heart diseases, stomach disorders, breathing problems, weak *agni*, fevers
Onion	Hot, heavy, unctuous, pungent, sweet after digestion	Decreases *vata*, slightly increases *pitta , kapha*	Strengthening, increases semen
Coriander	Light, cold	Decreases *pitta*	Wholesome to heart and mind
Drumstick leaves	Hot, pungent	Decreases *vata, kapha*	Increases blood, used in treatments of spleen, edema, worms

Vegetables which are unseasonal, withered by the sun and winds, not cleaned properly and uncooked should not be consumed

Common name of the food	Qualities	Effects on Vitalities	Effects on various bodily processes
Fenugreek	Bitter, hot, pungent after digestion	Pacifies *vata*, increases *pitta*, destroys *kapha*	Good for diabetics, reduces fat
Spinach	Cold, heavy, little pungent, sweet	Increases *vata*, *kapha*	Not to be taken in blood disorders
Mushroom	Cold, slimy, astringent, heavy, sweet	Increases *vata*, *pitta*, *kapha*	Strength giving
Mutton	Light, unctuous, sweet after digestion, cold	Pacifies *vata*, *pitta*, *kapha*	Builds strength, bulk promoting, increases virility
Lamb	Very light	Pacifies *vata*, *pitta*, *kapha*	Gives strength to heart
Beef	Very heavy	Increase *Pitta*, *kapha*	Unwholesome
Pork	Heavy, hot, unctuous, sweet	Pacifies *vata*, increases *pitta*, *kapha*	Promotes bulk
Shellfish	Cold, unctuous, sweet, sweet after digestion	Decreases *vata*, increases *pitta*	Strength giving, Increase feces in the body

Common name of the food	Qualities	Effects on Vitalities	Effects on various bodily processes
Old meat	Unwholesome	Vitiate *vata, pitta, kapha*	Causes several diseases
Fish	Sweet, hot, heavy, unctuous, sweet after digestion	Decreases *vata*, increases *pitta, kapha*	Strengthening, nourishing; avoid combining with milk.
Fish eggs	Unctuous	Increase *kapha*	Nourishing, but may can cause dyspepsia
Chicken	Unctuous, heavy, hot, astringent	Pacifies *vata*	Nourishing, strength giving,
Eggs	Very unctuous, heavy, sweet, sweet after digestion	Pacifies *vata*	Nourishing, increase semen
Milk	Sweet, unctuous, cold, heavy, sweet after digestion	Pacifies *vata, pitta* Increases *kapha*	Life sustaining, nourishing, build bodily tissues and *ojas*, enhances virility
Cow's milk	Sweet, heavy, cold, slimy	Pacifies *vata, pitta*	Very nourishing, cures heart burns, increases breast milk, cures anaemia
Goat's milk	Cold, light, astringent, sweet	Pacifies *vata, pitta, kapha*	Strengthen digestive fire, constipating, used in fevers, coughs

Stale or old meat should not be consumed.

Common name of the food	Qualities	Effects on Vitalities	Effects on various bodily processes
Fresh yogurt	Heavy, hot, sweet, astringent, unctuous, sour after digestion	Increases *pitta, kapha*	Promotes appetite, strength giving, used in diarrhea, nasal diseases, not to be used in conditions of oedema in the body
Whey *(water of fresh yogurt)*	Light	Moves *doshas*	Cleanses body channels, nourishes
Butter milk *with water, without fat*	Light, cold, sweet, dry, sour, sweet after digestion	Pacifies *vata, pitta, kapha*	Wholesome, digestive, used in urinary obstructions, piles
Seasame oil	Heavy, subtle, sweet, hot, astringent as a secondary taste, sweet after digestion	Decreases *vata, kapha* Increases *pitta*	Spreads fast (*vyavayi*),acts immediately (*vikashi*) strengthens body, prepared with herbs helps in curing many diseases
Mustard oil	Light, hot, pungent, bitter, pungent after digestion	Decreases *vata, kapha* Vitiates *pitta*	Used in excess can cause blood disorders. Decreases fats, semen
Safflower oil	Sour, hot, heavy	Increases *pitta, kapha*	
Castor oil	Hot, slimy, heavy, subtle, bitter, pungent, sweet after digestion	Pacifies *vata*	Causes thirst, helps digestion, reduces stomach distension, swelling

Common name of the food	Qualities	Effects on Vitalities	Effects on various bodily processes
Almond oil	Hot, light	Controls *kapha*	Nourishing qualities
Groundnut oil	Sweet, cold, unctuous, heavy, sweet after digestion	Increases *vata, kapha*	
Sunflower oil	Bitter, salty, pungent, sweet, cold in potency, dry, heavy, alkaline, sweet after digestion	Increases *vata, pitta* Decreases *kapha*	Helps easy expulsion of the wastes from the body
Corn oil	Sweet, cold, dry, heavy, sweet after digestion	Increases *vata* Controls *pitta, kapha*	Constipating, used in blood disorders
Coconut oil	Heavy	Controls *vata, pitta*	
Honey	Cold, light, dry, subtle, sweet, astringent	Decreases *vata, pitta* very slightly Destroys *kapha*	Enhances the qualities of the substance with which gets mixed
Sugarcane juice	Sweet, cold, unctuous	Decreases *vata, pitta*	Moves wastes from the body
Jaggery (gud)	Sweet, hot, unctuous	Controls *vata*	Moves wastes from the body, nourishes
Coconut (fruit)	Cold, heavy, unctuous, sweet, sweet after digestion	Decreases *vata, pitta* Increases *kapha*	Causes constipation

Common name of the food	Qualities	Effects on Vitalities	Effects on various bodily processes
Grapes	Cold, unctuous, sweet, sour, astringent, heavy, sweet after digestion	Decreases *vata, pitta* Increases *kapha*	Helps formation and excretion of urine and feces
Raisins	Sweet, sweet after digestion	Destroys *vata*	
Gooseberry	Cold, dry, sweet after digestion	Pacifies *vata, pitta, kapha*	Good for eyes, brain and digestion
Custard apple	Sweet, cold, sweet after digestion	Decreases *vata, pitta* Increases *kapha*	Increases formation of blood
Pineapple	Sweet, heavy	Increases *pitta*	
Banana *(ripe)*	Heavy, cold, unctuous, sweet	Destroys *pitta* Increases *kapha*	Quenches thirst. Used in blood disorders
Lemon	Light, sour, pungent, astringent	Pacifies *vata, pitta, kapha*	
Guava	Cold, heavy, sour, astringent		
Pomegranate	Light, unctuous, cold, sweet, astringent as secondary taste	Pacifies *vata, pitta kapha*	Gives strength to the heart

Common name of the food	Qualities	Effects on Vitalities	Effects on various bodily processes
Mango (ripe)	Unctuous, heavy, sweet, astringent	Decreases *vata* Increases *kapha*	Ignites *agni*, gives strength
Date	Cold, unctuous, heavy, sweet, sweet after digestion	Destroys *vata*	Strength giving, can cause constipation
Almonds	Unctuous, hot, sweet	Decreases *vata, pitta*	Strength giving, to be avoided in *pitta* diorders
Apple	Heavy, cold, sweet, sweet after digestion	Increases *kapha*	Promotes bulk
Orange	Hot, heavy, sweet, sour	Decreases *vata*, increases *pitta, kapha*	Strength giving
Blueberries	Dry, hot, sweet astringent	Pacifies *vata, pitta, kapha*	Used in curing disorders of blood, controlling blood sugar level
Ginger	Heavy, hot, dry, pungent, sweet after digestion	Destroys *vata, kapha*	Excellent digestive, used in treating most of the disorders of *vata, pitta,* and *kapha*

Spices

Spices not only enhance the flavour of the food, they also transform qualities of the food. They assist in increasing digestion and metabolism. Most spices are pungent and warming. Some decrease *kapha* (binder) and heaviness, others decrease *vata* (mover) and increase *pitta* (transformer).

For instance, with proper spices, one can change the heavier foods or foods which are high in nutrition but are dense (fats, meats, desserts, wheat preparations) into more digestible foods otherwise they will lead to excess heaviness in the body and clog of the channels.

It is preferable to buy whole spices and grind them when required. Since it is difficult for everyone to do this, the next best solution is to grind them on a weekly basis and keep them in airtight containers and away from sunlight.

Spices need to be sautéed in oil or dry roasted before use. Normally seeds are the first to be sautéed and powders are added only later on.

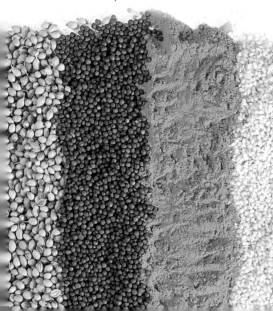
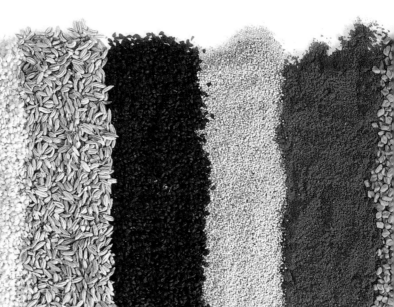

Substance SPICES		Taste and qualities	Heating or cooling	Post Digestive Effect	Effects on Three *Doshas*	Therapeutic value
Heeng (H) *Ferula asafetida (B)*	ASAFOETIDA	Pungent	Heating	Pungent light, unctuous	Decreases *vata & kapha.* Increases *pitta*	Digestive, strengthens *agni*, expels *ama.,* used in treating flatulence, abdominal distension respiratory disorders, given extensively post delivery to keep *vata* in balance.
Kali Mirch (H)	BLACK PEPPER	Pungent light; dry, rough	Heating	Pungent	Increases *Pitta,* Stimulates *Vata.* Decreases *Kapha.*	Promotes digestion, can cross blood brain barrier, carries nutrition to the brain
Ela (small) *Elaichi*	CARDAMOM	Pungent Light, bitter, hot	Heating	Sweet	Taken in excess can increase *pitta.* Relieves *vata & kapha.*	Promotes digestion Relieves nausea, reduces mucus effect when added to sweet milk desserts
Ajamoda *Ajwan (H)*	CAROM SEED OR BISHOP'S WEED	Pungent, Light, bitter	Heating	Pungent	Increases *pitta,* Decreases *vata & kapha.*	Treats digestive disorders, is antispasmodic in colic and relieves flatulence
Twak(S) *Dalchini (H)* *Cinnamomum zeylanicum (B)*	CINNAMON	Sweet, pungent, astringent	Heating	Sweet	Decreases *kapha & pitta* (not to be used in any bleeding disorder)	Carries nutrition to the tissues, relieves thirst and dryness of mouth. Helps digesting heavy, sweet foods, used in treating sinus congestion, bronchitis
Lavanga (S) *Caryophyllus aromaticus (B)*	CLOVE	Pungent	Heating	Pungent	Increases *pitta,* decreases *vata & kapha.*	Stimulant, improves *agni,* expectorant, used in cold, cough, toothache, lends aroma to food

S - S A N S K R I T,   B - B O T A N I C A L,   H - H I N D I

Substance SPICES		Taste and qualities	Heating or cooling	Post Digestive Effect	Effects on Three *Doshas*	Therapeutic value
Dhania (H) *Coriandrum* *sativum (B)*	CORIANDER SEED	Seed dry, light	Cooling	Sweet	Stimulates *vata* & *kapha*, Relieves *Pitta.* (to be used sparingly in bronchial conditions)	Digestive, treats indigestion nausea, dysentery very useful in relieving acidity, relieves burning sensation while passing urine, good diuretic
Jeera (H) *Cuminum* *cyminum (B)*	BLACK CUMIN	Pungent hot, light, dry	Heating	Pungent	Decreases *vata* & *kapha.* Stimulates *pitta*	Digestive, treats diarrhea, piles, improves breast milk secretion,
Methi (H) (S) *Trigonella* *foenumgraeceum (B)*	FENUGREEK (SEED)	Pungent hot, light, dry	Heating	Pungent	Decreases *vata* & *kapha* ,stimulates *pitta* (not to be used during pregnancy and in *pitta* disorders)	promotes digestion, aphrodisiac, diuretic, rejuvenates, used in uterus cleansing after child birth
Saunf (H) *Shatpushpa (S)* *Foeniculum* *vulgaris (B)*	FENNEL SEED	Unctuous, Sweet, Hot	Heating	Pungent	Decreases *vata, kapha*	Best digestive, strengthens *agni,* calming to the nerves, diuretic, removes phlegm in bronchial conditions, freshens the breath, its decoction helps in relieving sleeplessness.
Shunddhi (S)	GINGER (DRY POWDER)	Pungent Heavy, Dry, Rough	Heating	Sweet	Relieves *vata* & *kapha.* Stimulates *Pitta*	Stimulates *agni,* helps digestion, dry powder massage helps relieve joint pains. A must-have spice in rainy season
Jatiphala (S) *Jaiphal (H)* *Myristica* *fragrans (B)*	NUTMEG	Pungent Bitter, astringent, hot, dry, light	Heating	Pungent	Decreases *vata* & *kapha..* Increases *pitta* (very potent, to be used in very small quantity and	Stimulant, aphrodisiac, Used in treating poor absorption or wasting diseases, cough, intestinal worms, skin conditions like

110

Substance SPICES		Taste and qualities	Heating or cooling	Post Digestive Effect	Effects on Three *Doshas*	Therapeutic value
					sparingly, can produce instant burning in stomach, vomiting, giddiness)	acne and eczema.
Kesar (H) *Crocus sativus (B)*	SAFFRON	Pungent, unctuous, astringent, hot	Cooling	Sweet	Neutralizes three *doshas*, can stimulate all the *doshas* if used excessively.	Strengthens all the tissues, special effect on reproductive tissues, Helps digestion and assimilation of heavy and nourishing diets, Enhances complexion.
Saindha namak	SALT	Salty heavy, rough	Heating	Sweet	Relieves *vata.*, increases *pitta*, *kapha*,	Powerful stimulant, digestive, should be cooked along with the food and not sprinkled, Excess use leads to wrinkles, greying of hair, water retention and bone loss.
Til *Gingely* *Sesamum indicum*	SESAME (SEED)	Sweet, bitter & astringent	Heating	Pungent	Heavy, oily, smooth, strengthening. Increases *pitta* & *kapha*, Decreases *vata.*	
Haldi (H) *Haridra (S)* *Curcuma longa (B)*	TURMERIC	Bitter, pungent & astringent	Heating	Pungent	Increases *vata* & *pitta*, relieves *kapha*	Cleanses all tissue-elements in the body, has a drying effect on mucus, given in internal injuries, it is anti-inflammatory, antiseptic and antibacterial Helps in diabetes, promotes digestion, enhances complexion.

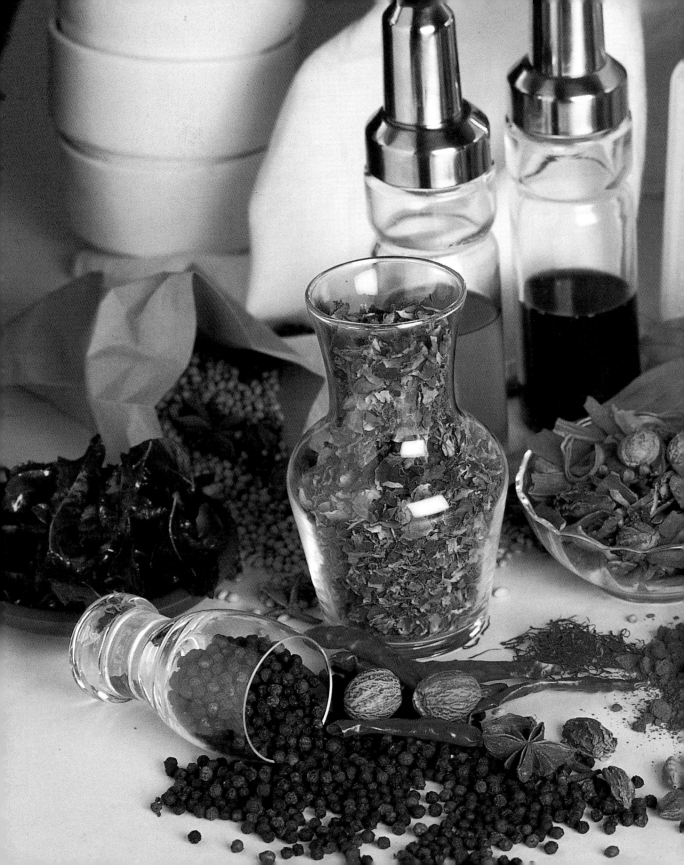

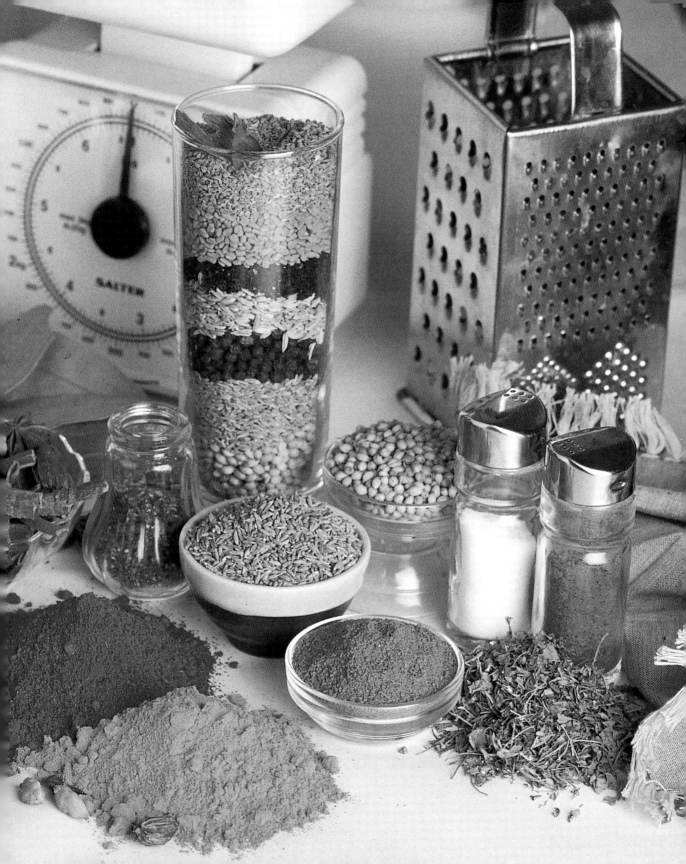

Dietics

~

Ayurveda deals extensively with food and has a rationale for creating food patterns required to suit the bodily well being of each individual according to his/her particular constitution.

Ayurvedic text clearly states that 'a self controlled person should take food only after considering the seven factors related to food which are: *svabhava* (natural qualities or nature of food), *samyoga* (mixture or food combinations), *samskara* (preparing, cooking, processing), *matra* (quantity), *desa* (habitat or body), *kala* (time of the day, season/ age of the individual or stage of the disease) and *upayoga vyavastha* (mode of using). These are the common causes of health or ill health.

Due consideration needs to be given to each of these factors to enable better digestion and better health.

1. Nature of food: One has to know the nature of food and the inherent qualities by which the food substances act on the body. For instance, ginger is digestive, coriander is cooling and jaggery (*gud*) is nourishing. However, these natural qualities of foods can change depending on how they are prepared or combined with other food substances.

2. The combination of two or more substances can bring about a change in the nature of substances thus combined. The resultant attribute does not originally belong to the individual constituent. For instance, puffed rice is light but becomes heavy when combined with milk.

3. *Samskara* or processing by a particular method can transform the inherent qualities of the food substances.

Ayurveda lists these procedures as
    (a) contact with water, dilution, adding water
    (b) contact with fire, all kinds of application of heat
    (c) cleaning or washing
    (d) churning
    (e) place of storage
    (f) time (maturing)
    (g) flavouring
    (h) impregnation
    (i) presentation
    (j) vessel or container used.

On a daily basis, we can observe these processes and see how they bring about changes in the foods we consume. For instance, yogurt is hard to digest but when we put water and churn it to make buttermilk or lassi, it becomes very light. Water kept overnight in a silver container becomes an immunity enhancer.

4. *Matra* is the quantity of food to be taken. As a rule, the quantity of the food is decided according to the nature of *agni* (fire) and heaviness or lightness (vis-à-vis digestion) of the food substances. The quantity of the food differs from individual to individual. It takes into consideration age, constitution, sex and power of digestion.

Improper quantity is of two types:

(a) Quantitative dietary deficiency (*hinamatra*), includes under-nutrition due to insufficient food. It can lead to reduced bodily strength, mental strength, and power of sense organs. Decline in *ojas*, impairment of body tissues, *vata* (mover) disorders and result in ill health.

(b) Quantitative over-nutrition (*atimatra*) eating more than the capacity and requirement of the body leads to vitiation of all the *doshas*. Imbalanced *vata* (mover) creates colic pain, fainting, obstructs channels. *Pitta* (transformer) causes fever, thirst, burning sensation, delirium, and diarrhea. *Kapha* (binder) causes vomiting, indigestion, accumulation of *ama* and heaviness of the body.

5. *Desa* refers to both the region in which the food substance is grown and also to the region where the consumer lives. Habitat determines the qualities of the foods due to the role of land, water, winds and the nature of the climate in which the substance grows.

    Desa also refers to the body of the user, like the state of health, constitution and digestive capacity.

incorrect food combinations

Various kinds of foods, when eaten together, make our digestive system secrete many different digestive enzymes simultaneously, making the process of digestion a difficult task. Undigested food clogs the intestines, ferments, putrefies and eventually build up toxins in the body. It is best to take the foods which do not combine well at different times of the day or at different meals. Given below are some examples of incorrect food combinations. According to Ayurveda, these combinations, if persisted in dietary habits, create vitiation of *doshas*, bodily tissues *(dhatus)* and bodily wastes.

~ Milk followed by fruits and vice versa

~ Taking sour substances like bread (fermented with yeast) along with milk.

~ Milk with salt

~ Milk with meat of any kind

~ Clarified butter kept in a bronze vessel

~ Hot drinks after alcohol, yogurt or honey

~ Cold and hot substances together

~ Cold water after a hot meal

~ Honey in hot water

~ Banana with milk, yogurt or buttermilk

~ Chicken with yogurt

~ Fish with sugar

~ Cucumber or tomatoes with lemon.

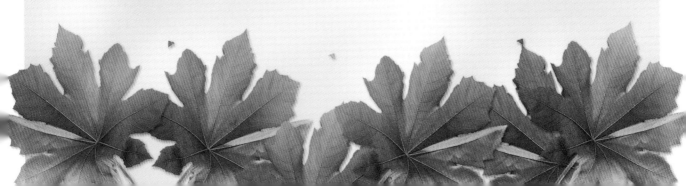

6. *Kala* refers to various time periods like time of the day or night, time of the year or seasons according to which the choice of food has to be made. Time also refers to the age of the person and the stage of the disease (if it exists) in due accordance to which the food has to be taken.

7. *Upayoga vyavastha* refers to the manner of taking food or dietetic rules. We will deal with them in more detail.

8. *Upyoktrin,* the food habit of the individual.

Incompatible Diet *(Viruddha Ahara)*

Ayurveda gives us a unique concept of an incompatible diet. According to Ayurveda, any substance either as food or medicine which provokes the *dosha* in the body but does not expel the substance out of it, is regarded as unwholesome. When *doshas* remain in the body, aided by an unhealthy diet, they become causal factors for diseases in the body. Even if one knows the nature and functions of the dietary substances, it is not a complete knowledge. One also has to know how a particular substance acts in combination with other substances and what kind of transformation it undergoes when it is combined with other substances or processed.

Ayurveda provides us with the details of substance incompatibility due to their variance with place, time, digestive power, dosage, habit, *doshas,* mode of preparation, potency, state of health, order, proscription and prescription, cooking, combination, palatability and rules of dietetics. It is considered a serious violation of healthy living if one fails to avoid the incompatible choices.

Disorders and diseases like inflammation, dropsy, jaundice, abscesses in the body, ulcers in the stomach and many other pathological conditions can erupt due to an incompatible diet. It can also lead to depletion of strength, vigour and memory.

1. **Incompatibility with place or region:** Food that has similar qualities to the climate in which it is eaten is incompatible to that region. For instance, in a is humid area, a regular diet which is heavy, cold and moist, will produce diseases of *kapha* (binder). Similarly, having dry and tart substances in dry regions is not recommended.

2. **Seasonal incompatibility:** Having cold, dry and light foods in winter is incompatible with the season, since it will vitiate *vata* (mover) and the digestive fires, which during this season require sweet, sour and salty dietary intake. Similarly, a hot and pungent diet in summer is harmful For people who move from place to place where seasons differ, it is advisable to modify their diet accordingly.

3. **Incompatible with digestive power:** If the digestion is sluggish eating large heavy meals is contrary to digestion. Having a heavy meal after a period of fasting, not eating at the proper time and eating less when very hungry are examples of behaviour to digestion.

4. **Incompatibility with the proportion or dosage:** Some substances are incompatible because of their proportion. The most cited example is that of honey and clarified butter (*ghee*), which is toxic if mixed together in equal quantity. In this proportion they vitiate *doshas* and body tissues.

5. **Incompatibility of *dosha*:** Food, which is similar to the individual's constitution is incompatible to the dominant *dosha* of the person. Since Ayurveda works on the principle of similar increases and dissimilar decreases, if a person of a *vata* (mover) constitution takes a dry, bitter and rough diet, which is predominantly a *vata* (mover) diet, he will have a *vata* imbalance. Similarly, if a *kapha* (binder) person takes a *kapha* diet, it is incompatible with his particular *dosha*.

6. **Incorrect method of preparation:** Sometimes the preparation of a particular substance is incompatible with the health of the body. For instance, eating improperly set yogurt; fish cooked in linseed oil, and meat cooked in a copper vessel are some of the examples of incompatibility. Honey should never be cooked. Uncooked honey is nectar; cooked honey is poison. Ayurveda considers uncooked. overcooked or burnt foods incompatible and unwholesome.

7. **Incompatibilities with potency:** Substances that have a cooling potency are incompatible with substances having hot potency. Combining fish with milk is incompatible. Having fruits like apple, pineapple with milk is incompatible.

8. **Incompatibility with bowel habits:** In case of difficult bowel movements, a diet of pulses, uncooked or raw green vegetables and roots would be inadvisable. Such a diet will lead to *vata* (mover) imbalance and bind the wastes, which can cause piles and various similar diseases.

9. **Incompatibility with the state of health:** Eating food that has vitiating qualities vis-à-vis the state of health of a person is incompatible. Taking a *vata* (mover) inducing diet after physical

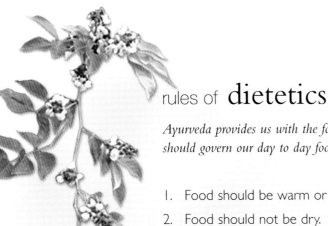

rules of dietetics

Ayurveda provides us with the following principles, which should govern our day to day food regimen

1. Food should be warm or hot.
2. Food should not be dry.
3. Food has to be taken in proper quantities.
4. Food should only be taken again, when the previous meal is digested.
5. Food taken should not be contradictory in their potency.
6. Food should be taken in a proper place with required accessories.
7. Food should not be eaten in a hurry.
8. The process of intake should not be exceedingly slow.
9. While eating, concentrate on food properly.
10. Only that food should be taken which is wholesome to the individual's physical constitution and psychic temperament.
11. For the purpose of taking food, Ayurveda divides the capacity of the stomach into three. One part is filled with solids, the second part with liquids and the third part is left for the movement of the three *doshas*. There should be:
    (a) No undue pressure on the stomach;
    (b) No obstruction in the proper functioning of the heart;
    (c) No pressure on the sides of the chest;
    (d) No heaviness in the abdomen;
    (e) A feeling that the senses have been properly nourished;
    (f) Relief from hunger and thirst;
    (g) A feeling of comfort in such activities like standing, sitting, walking, sleeping, laughing, inhaling and exhaling;
12. Food taken in the morning should be digested by evening and food taken in the evening should be digested by next morning;
13. There should be an increase in bodily strength, good complexion and well-being

exhaustion or sexual activity. These activities are *vata* governed; inducing more of this vitality would tend to vitiate it.

10. **Incorrect order:** Ayurveda gives due importance to the order of dietetics. One is not supposed to consume food before emptying the bladder and bowel. It also means the order in which food is to be taken. Food should start with sweet substances, (*agni* being strong in the beginning, it can digest sweets easily), then one can have food having *amla* (digestive and salivary secretion) and *lavana rasa* (appetizer, moistening) and at the end, *tikta* (mouth cleaning), *kashaya* (decreasing salivary secretion) products can be consumed. This also refers to avoiding or adhering to norms by which certain foods need to be taken.

11. **Incompatibility of combination:** Certain food, when combined, become incompatible and unwholesome (see box).

12. **Incompatibility with rules of dietetics:** If one does not follow rules of taking food, there is an incompatibility with the method.

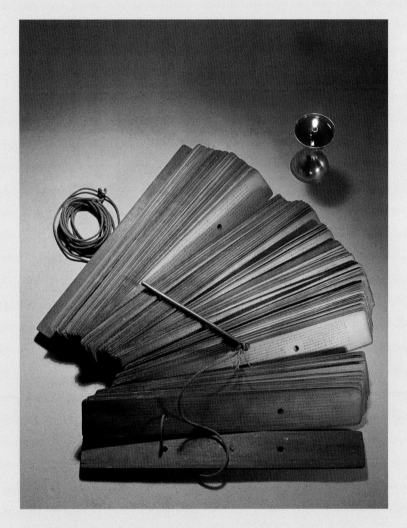

The *Caraka Samhita*, the most significant text on the diagnosis and treatment of disease in Ayurveda, emphasizes the importance of a healthy diet – if a person is eating a wholesome diet, he will not need any medicine, and if his diet is faulty, no medicine can help him.

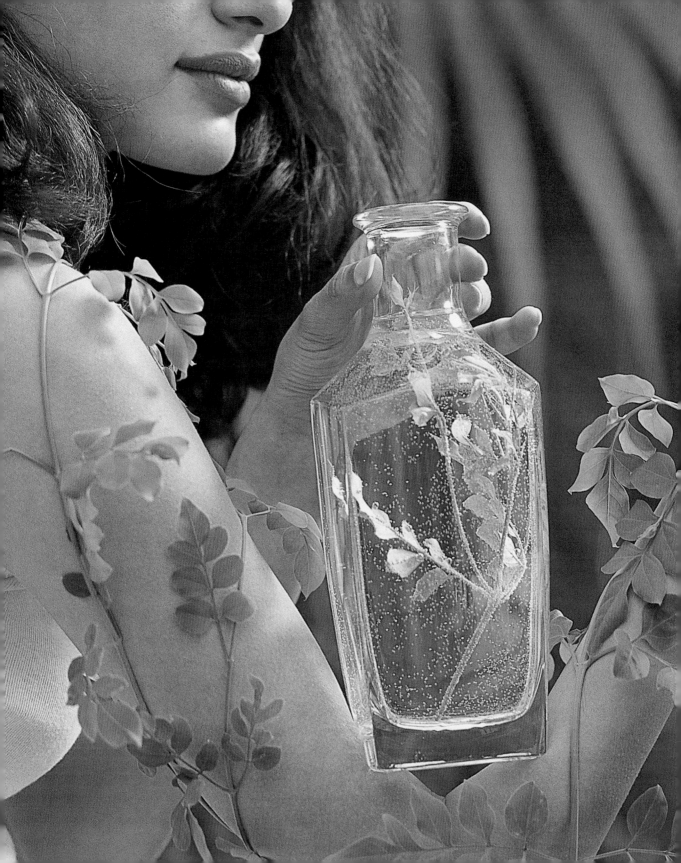

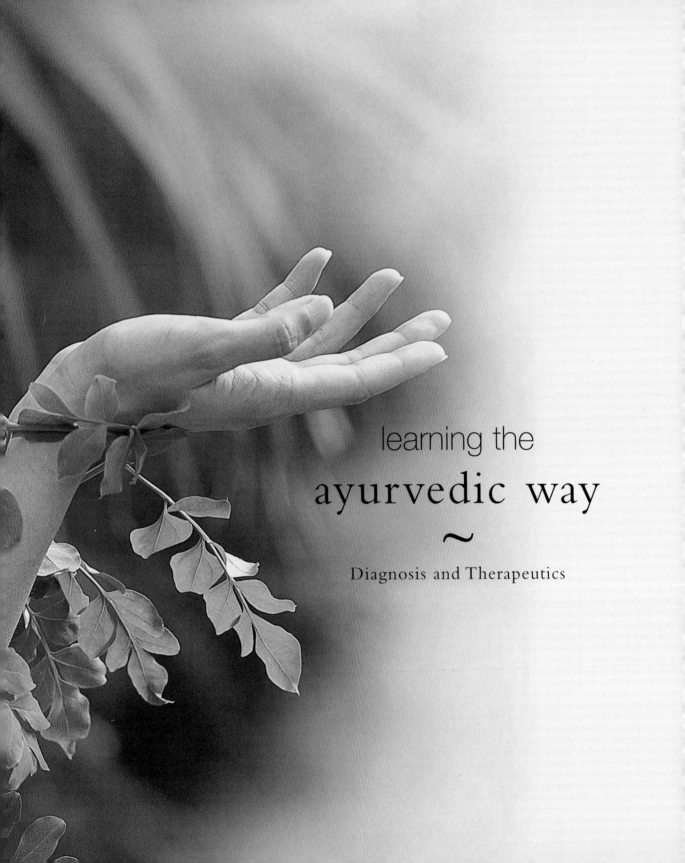

learning the
ayurvedic way
~

Diagnosis and Therapeutics

D iagnosis in Ayurveda is detailed, intensive and extensive. Diagnosis is multi-fold as it takes into account the bodily constitution, the psychic constitution and the age of the patient, the patient's pathological conditions, vitality of the bodily tissues the body's structure and its measures are observed. The capacity to digest food and to exert are also important points to be looked into. The purpose of this examination is to assess the strength of the patient and the intensity of the disorder so as to determine the course of therapy.

At the physical level, the examination looks at the pulse, tongue, eyes, voice, urine, stool, skin and the over all appearance of the patient. These are significant indicators of the nature and the state of the bodily imbalance.

Sensitivity towards one's own body structure and functioning can warn the person of an impending disease. Advance knowledge of these signs and symptoms is one of the strongest points in Ayurvedic diagnostics. Bodily self-awareness can equip the person to take corrective measures before early symptoms take root in the body, in the form of a disease. Most of the early symptoms of bodily disorders are self-limiting. At this stage, an appropriate intervention can help the body to regain its balance.

Sensitivity towards one's own body
structure and functioning can warn the
person of an impending disease.
Advance knowledge of these signs
and symptoms is one of the strongest
points in Ayurvedic diagnostics.

Major factors which contribute to the presence of disease in the body are the

- imbalance of *vata, pitta* and *kapha*
- vitiation of the body tissues (*dhatus*) and the body wastes (*malas*)
- weak digestive power
- undigested food material (*ama*)
- and vitiated state of bodily channels (*srotas*)

The major causes of all diseases have been classified in three categories:

1. Improper conjunction of the senses with surrounding objects causes various ailments. This can be in the form of non-use, excessive or improper use of the sense organs. Reading in poor light, over exposure to loud noise, excessive intake of food of a particular taste, and an unsanitary lifestyle are some examples of the inappropriate use of senses vis-à-vis their objects.

2. Change of seasons or other changes in time and space can cause ailments if we are not prepared for it or do not adapt to it. Seasonal changes, or change of living place can become causal factors of diseases.

3. When people make wrong decisions and wrong choices (affecting their health) due to impaired intellect and stress they fall ill. Not following healthy habits, taking food contrary to one's constitution and negative thoughts are some of the examples of a misuse of intellect.

Digestion – the power of *Agni*

It is apparent, that for Ayurveda, diet and digestion hold the key to health.

According to Ayurveda, equal care of both is essential for maintaining good health. Choosing an improper diet for one's particular constitution can lead to imbalances and following improper dietary habits can weaken and hamper digestion. Whereas well-digested and well-chosen foods would create health and well being, improper digestion can turn food into *ama* or toxins in one's body.

When food is digested properly, the body is able to reap the nutritional benefit from the ingested food; it becomes strong and energetic. Contrary to this, when there is indigestion or any other problem at any level of the digestive process, the immediate effect is seen in bodily fatigue, loss of energy, non-specific pains and aches, lethargy or simply a lack of vigour.

A weak digestion becomes the root cause of all the ills that can ail the body, since food is not properly digested by the digestive fire; thus, it can neither nourish the bodily tissues (*dhatus*) nor develop them. A weak body becomes a host to a myriad of diseases. Ayurveda has dealt with the phenomena of digestion, indigestion and disorders related to bad digestion in a major way.

Here, we shall deal with most common of the digestive disorders, which can be diagnosed and treated by a discerning and perceptive individual.

Ayurveda holds digestive fire to be of four types:

1. Weak fire (where the digestive fire is sluggish)
2. Strong digestive fire (it is intense and can digest anything).
3. Irregular or erratic digestive fire (it is sometimes weak and at other times strong)
4. Balanced digestive fire (functions normally in the body). It is normal with respect to the individual body type.

We will be concerned here with weak digestive fire, which, if remains untreated, can become the cause of many other diseases in the body.

It is vitally important not to put more burden on an already weak digestion. Kindling the digestive fire is of utmost importance for a healthy life span. Eating only when hungry, taking easily digestible food, using digestion enhancing herbs like ginger, *pippali*, black pepper, cinnamon, *trikatu* and *triphala;* adding spices like cumin, coriander, asafoetida and fennel seeds to daily meals (one can also make tea of a chosen spice and drink it after the meal); observing a weekly fast and doing body specific exercises – all these help strengthen the bodily fires and aid in the process of digestion.

Indigestion

Ayurveda considers indigestion or dyspepsia, a disorder of weak digestive powers, which can be easily avoided if one follows some rules of dietetics. In general, there are several causal factors, which

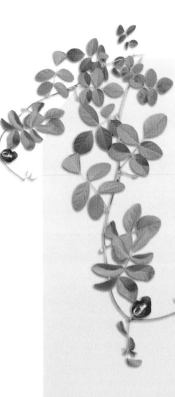

the five fires

There are five kinds of fire (*agni* and *igneous* have same linguistic roots) in every person –

1. **Digestive fires (jataragni)**, from mouth to anus (especially the stomach and small intestine), transform food to nutritive essences (*ahara rasa*);
2. **Metabolic fires (ranjakagni)**, in the liver, spleen and stomach, transforms nutritive essences to enzymes for body tissues (*dhatu*s);
3. **Apparitional fires (sadhakagni)**, especially in the heart, is responsible for memory and other mental functions;
4. **Sight fires (alocakagni)**, in visual sense organs, are responsible for vision and the sparkle in the eyes;
5. **Absorption fires (bhrajakagni)**, in the skin and lungs, responsible for the lustre of skin.

In fact, these five fires are sub-types of transformer vital functions. Amongst these, the digestive and metabolic fires are important for processing food in the body.

Digestive and metabolic fires transform food into forms of

matter useful for the body and into residual waste products (*ama*). These wastes, if not excreted out of the body, become toxins. If there is a disturbance in the functions of fire, for instance if the fires become weak, there is an excess production of undigested residue or non-production of nutritive essences.

Ayurveda has looked carefully at these processes in terms of desirable or undesirable influx of matter under different conditions of the body. Since the influx of matter is controllable as a diet or drug, various conditions of the body can be addressed by appropriately designing influx to suit the condition. Ayurvedic reasoning is based on the qualities of substances, their transformations and their potency.

Once the digestive process is complete, nutritional essences are the products. These products are found to have post-digestive effects. They are either sweet or sour or pungent. Saline, bitter and astringent tastes are never found dominant in the nutritive essences into which the food transforms. Metabolic fires transform nutritive essences eventually into tissues. The changes occur because metabolic fires can be influenced if the original diet/drug matter has the power to affect sweet, sour or pungent essences. These essences are known as *vipaka,* or after-taste.

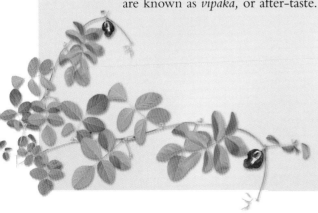

can lead to indigestion; one has to determine the specific cause or causes according to the individual .

General causes:

- ▶ Weak digestive power.
- ▶ Eating to the fullest capacity of the stomach.
- ▶ Eating too fast.
- ▶ Eating before the previous meal is digested.
- ▶ Regular intake of heavy foods.
- ▶ Taking more fats and oils than required.
- ▶ Regular consumption of hot and spicy food.
- ▶ Contaminated water.
- ▶ Drinking cold water or drinks after hot food.
- ▶ Intestinal worms.
- ▶ Eating incompatible foods.
- ▶ Any systemic imbalance i.e. inflammation or ulceration of the stomach or liver malfunctioning etc.
- ▶ Vitiation of *vata, pitta* and *kapha.*

Symptoms

There is a feeling of discomfort in the stomach region, a sense of abdominal bloating, loss of appetite, coated tongue, nausea, pain in the legs, acid reflux, stomachache and a general malaise.

Treatment

Eat as little as possible till symptoms of indigestion disappear. Take light and easily digestible food only. Clear vegetable soups and gruel helps to kindle digestive fire. Try to follow the rules of dietetics.

Take half a teaspoon of roasted bishop's weed (*ajwain*) with a pinch of rock salt, drink warm water after that. It relieves flatulence, stomach ache and distended stomach.

Drink buttermilk after meals; add roasted cumin seed powder, dry mint powder, rock salt and black pepper to the drink. It takes care of loss of appetite and aids digestion.

Apply a small grain of asafoetida dissolved in warm water all over the abdomen to cure colic amongst infants. This is also an effective remedy for non-specific stomach pain in children.

Chew a piece of ginger with lemon and rock salt before the meal to rekindle the digestive fire.

De-stress your body. Stress, whether emotional or mental, gets stored in the stomach, making all remedies loose their efficacy.

Constipation

In this condition a regular bowel movement is restricted. Evacuation waste from the colon becomes difficult or irregular. The accumulation of the waste in intestines leads to putrefaction and flatulence. The body cannot handle constipation for a long time without showing symptoms of discomfort or disease. Some of the symptoms which the body manifests singly or in combination are: lack of the urge to pass the stool, a coated tongue, foul breath, loss of appetite, headaches, acidity, dark circles under the eyes; heaviness in the abdomen, pain in the lumbar region, mouth ulcers and general lethargy. Chronic constipation can cause various bodily dispositions like high blood pressure, joint pains and piles.

Causes

If there is no systemic obstruction in the body to expel stool, improper food habits is the major cause of constipation. Habitual intakes of cold, heavy, excessively spiced, dry and rough (non lubricating) foods invariably cause constipation. The modern fad of excluding all possible fats from the diet for a normal person tends to vitiate *vata*. Irregular eating habits, intake of incompatible foods, insufficient intake of water and drinking very cold water after the meal bind the feces. Lack of physical activity and emotional distress can also cause constipation.

Treatment

Changing the diet is a major step toward treating constipation. One has to first relieve constipation and then go on a light, easy to digest diet for some days, to decongest the digestive passage.

Haritaki (*Terminalia chebula*) *Isabgole* (*phyllium husk*) Senna leaves (*Cassia angustifolia*) are some of the choicest herbs to ease out the difficult stool from the body; a powder of either one or both can be tried. Figs or raisins can be soaked in water overnight in a non-metallic container. Soak two to three figs or ten raisins in a glass of water. Drink the water it is soaked in, and eat the fruit. *Triphala* is another remedy for relieving constipation. Soak a teaspoon of *triphala* powder in water in a nonmetallic glass overnight and drink the water after straining it.

Diarrhea

The symptoms differ according to the different *dosha* imbalances. It is important to know the cause to have an effective treatment.

Preceding Symptoms

Some symptoms singly or in combination with others may get manifested before the onset of diarrhea.

Symptoms include distended stomach, indigestion, acidic reflux, nausea, or a piercing pain in the stomach.

Symptoms accompanying Diarrhea

Rumbling, heaviness of stomach, motions too often, dryness of mouth, thirst, pain in the calf muscle, burning sensation in the anus, loss of energy.

Kinds of diarrhea (atisara) and their symptoms

Vataja Diarrhea

Causes

Excess intake of rough, dry and deficient food, over indulgence in alcohol and sex, holding up the natural urges, excessive exposure to wind and sun and physical exercise beyond one's capacity. *Agni* weakens, the *vayu* gets vitiated and carries the fluids to colon to cause diarrhea.

Symptoms

Pain in the stomach, frequent, liquid stool, and rumbling in the stomach. Pain in the anus, thighs and lower back, dryness of mouth and increased respiration.

Pittaja Diarrhea

Causes

When a *pitta* person takes in excess sour, alkaline, pungent and salty food regularly. Exposure to scorching sun and hot winds, given to intense anger and envy. In such cases, his *pitta* gets vitiated, extinguishes his *agni* and reaches colon to liquefy the stool and causes diarrhea.

Symptoms

Excess thirst, burning sensation, sweat, stomach pain and inflammation of the anus.

Kaphaja Diarrhea

Causes

Large intake of heavy, sweet, cold and fatty substances. Heavy by nature and aided by cold and unctuousness, *kapha* extinguishes *agni* and due to its watery influence affects the colon to cause diarrhea.

Symptoms

The stool is heavy and mixed with mucus, it comes out in little quantity frequently. The person feels pain and heaviness in the abdomen, passes motion without knowledge. Nausea, aversion to food and lethargy are also symptoms.

Beside *vataj*, *pittaj* and *kaphaj* diarrhea, Ayurveda identifies a kind of diarrhea when all the three *doshas* are vitiated; it is the most serious variety. It can have, along with the above-mentioned symptoms, blood in stool. Fainting, fever and delirium can result from it.

This kind of diarrhea is caused by bad food, fear and anxiety. Ayurveda treats it under *vataj* diarrhea, since *vata* gets vitiated by fear and anxiety and treats accordingly by *vata* alleviating measures and providing happiness and consolation.

Treatment

Ayurveda advises against stopping the motion immediately, as the trapped feces will cause stiffness of body, piles, anemia, skin and stomach diseases and fever. The patient, however, has to be given fluids.

Consumption of buttermilk or whey is recommended. Whey is liquid portion of yogurt. Both liquids are beneficial in replacing the fluid loss and checking the diarrhea.

The dried rind of a pomegranate or inner peel of the rind of a pomegranate is a very effective remedy for diarrhea. A fine powder of dry rind or paste of fresh rind is to be taken with buttermilk.

Powdered coriander seeds can be taken with buttermilk four times a day.

A cool decocotion of boiled mint leaves can be taken two or three times a day.

Bael fruit (*aegle marmelos*) is one of the best remedies for curing diarrhea as well as bloody dysentery. Roast the unripe *bael* on fire and then take 3 to 4 grams of roasted pulp. The powder of dried *bael* is equally effective.

Diet

A light and liquid diet is recommended when suffering from diarrhea. Semi liquid rice gruel with fresh yogurt or puffed rice should be eaten. Buttermilk or a sweetened lemon drink (*sharbat*) can also be taken. Avoid foods heavy on digestion. It is also important to get a full night's sleep.

Commom Cold (*Pratisyaya*)

Ayurveda treats the common cold as a disorder of the nasal passage and nose. As a sense organ of smell, as a natural carrier of the air element in the body and above all, as a door to the brain, the nose is an extremely important organ of the body. As part of the nose care regimen, it is advised that we should not scratch it, nor remove hair from the inner walls of the nose – they filter the air that we breathe and protect the lungs.

medicinal food **buttermilk**

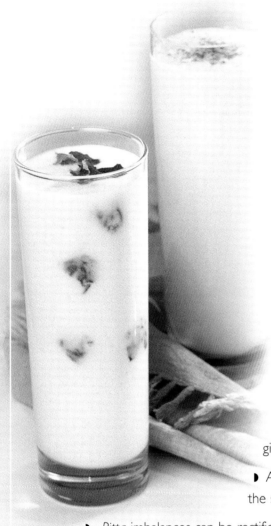

According to Ayurveda, buttermilk is the best liquid food for enhancing the digestive fire, and treating a number of disorders related to weak digestion.

It is prepared from churning fresh yogurt with water and removing the upper layer of butter from it. The remaining liquid is buttermilk.

This medicinal diet is wholesome when it is not thick, when it has been made of fresh curd and devoid of fat. It is sweet, sour and little astringent.

Buttermilk is helpful for people suffering from heaviness, anorexia, poor digestion, diarrhea and *vata/kapha/pitta* stomach disorders

‣ A person suffering from imbalance of all three *doshas* should take buttermilk with *trikatu* (powder of *pipali*, dry ginger and pepper) and salt.

‣ A person with *vata* imbalance in the stomach should have the same as above.

‣ *Pitta* imbalances can be rectified by sweet buttermilk adding sugar.

‣ In a *kapha* imbalance of the stomach, one should take buttermilk with all the fat removed, and mixed with rock salt, cumin seed powder, *trikatu* and honey.

‣ A person with an obstructed abdomen should take buttermilk with cumin(*jeera*) seeds and rock salt.

‣ A person with perforated abdomen should add honey to buttermilk.

‣ To be avoided when ailing from a cold, cough or suffering from acidity.

medicinal food honey

Ayurveda has called honey a food of the gods. It is healing, nourishing and also depletes *kapha*.

- Honey is cold in potency, dry, astringent in action and sweet in taste.
- Honey in general aggravates *vata* slightly; it is heavy, dry and rough, cold in potency and alleviates *pitta* as well as *kapha*.
- Since it is gathered from flowers of various kinds, having different qualities, tastes and potencies, it is considered to be highly therapeutic. Not only that, it also enhances the therapeutic properties of the drugs added to it.
- Honey is a cleanser of body channels. It is useful in skin problems, colds and coughs, obesity, thirst and difficulty in breathing. It is used both in constipation as well as diarrhea. It is good for the eyes and complexion. Ayurveda has classified honey into four categories:

    Maksika (honey collected from reddish type of honey bee)

    Bhramara (Honey collected from wasp type of bee)

    Ksaudra (honey collected from small bees.)

    Paittaka (honey collected from large bees)

- Out of these, honey from *maksika* bees is considered the best. *Maksika* type of honey is the color of sesame oil. *Paittaka* honey is the colour of *ghee*. *Ksaudra* honey is brown in colour and *bhramara* honey is white in colour.
- Honey should be taken in small quantities because it is heavy.
- Honey should neither be cooked, nor taken in hot water or any other hot drink like tea.
- According to Ayurveda, honey, if taken hot or if taken by a person exposed to heat, is fatal. This is because, during the collection process, it gets contaminated with poisonous material from the bees themselvs or from the various poisonous plants.
- Improper use of honey can bring harm to the body.

Symptoms

The most common symptoms of colds are heaviness in the head, a blocked or running nose, sneezing repeatedly, loss of taste, sore throat, congestion and sometimes accompanied by cough and body pain. The same common cold when left untreated for some time, shows symptoms of lightness of the head, discharge of dense mucus, change in voice and a feverish body.

Causes

Aggravation of *kapha* in the body, change of season, constipation, indigestion and accumulation of *ama* in the digestive track, intense anger, unnecessarily keeping awake late in the night.

Prolonged contact with cold-water and/or cold wind, exposure to cold or humid conditions and hot conditions alternatively within a short span of time also cause colds. Drinking ice-cold water or other drinks immediately after meals or coming from hot conditions can cause a common cold. Suppressing natural urges like vomiting, passing urine or waste, can also cause a cold.

Remedies

- Keep the head, ears, neck, chest and feet covered with warm clothes (if it is winter or windy).
- Boil fresh ginger and basil in water and drink it hot two or three times a day.
- Use more of ginger, honey, black pepper, cloves and cinnamon in daily food intake.
- Burn barley and inhale the fumes.
- Do not bathe in cold water.

- Do not sleep during the daytime.
- Having a thin soup of crab, chicken or mutton is therapeutic.
- Drink warm water.
- If the cold becomes chronic, take a paste of dry ginger, black pepper and honey in the morning.
- Take the juice out of leaves of basil (*tulsi*) and put two drops in each nostril.
- Take dry roasted chickepeas (*chana*), dry heat them, place them in a container near your nose and inhale the aroma before going to bed.
- For a sore throat, gargle with saline water twice or thrice a day to relieve irritation.
- For a dry cough, take half teaspoon of dry ginger powder, crystal sugar powder (*mishri*) with whey (yoghurt water) after meals.
- For a dry cough, make a paste of soaked, peeled and ground almonds (7 to 8) with half spoon of crystal sugar powder and white butter each. Divide it in three portions. Take it three times a day. Do not drink water after that.

Diet

Have barley, wheat and millet. Avoid rice. Take fenugreek, drumstick, bitter gourd and eggplant, as well as lentils. Take dates, papaya and black raisins. Avoid banana, guava, cucumber, all melons, pineapple or any sour fruit. Take ginger, garlic, onion, carrots, mint, coriander and radish. Avoid fried and stale food. Increase use of honey, turmeric, black pepper, cinnamon and hot water. Fasting also helps.

Doshas and Diseases

Ayurveda recognizes that the variation and the combination of diseases are almost countless. Diseases are seen as *processes* rather than *entities*. In this light, each disease needs to be understood keeping in mind these five factors: (a) cause of the disease; (b) early signs and symptoms; (c) the actual symptoms of the manifest disease; (d) exploratory therapy when one is unsure of the nature of disease (e) and the actual disease.

Vata, the most volatile of the three *doshas* moves *pitta* and *kapha.* When vitiated, *vata* is the main cause of inumerable diseases Many essential prescriptions of day and night regimen (waking, sleeping, oileation) revolve around keeping the *vata* in balance.

Here the classifications are only suggestive. However, some effort is made to provide a coherent picture vis-à-vis the criteria of classification and grouping of diseases.

Diseases are classified according to five different criteria. This is only one of the many kinds of classification, which are given in Ayurvedic texts:

Classification of Diseases & Disorders

Criteria of classification	Grouping of diseases	
Prognosis	Curable	Incurable
Intensity	Mild	Severe
Location	Mental	Physical
Nature of causative factors	Endogenous (internal to the body)	Exogenous (external to the body)
Site of origin	Originating from the stomach (*amasaya*). All diseases caused by aggravated *kapha* and *pitta* have their origin in the stomach.	Originates from the colon (*pakvasaya*). All diseases caused by aggravated *vata* has their origin in the colon.

Common Diseases & Disorders

Diseases of mover (*vata*)	Diseases of transformer (*pitta*)	Diseases of binder (*kapha*)
• Cracked nails, feet	• Heating, boiling, fuming	• Anorexia nervosa
• Pain and numbness of feet	• Acid eructation	• Drowsiness, excessive sleep
• Club foot, stiff ankle, cramps in the calf	• Burning sensation in chest	• Timidness
• Sciatica	• Burning sensation inside the body	• Heaviness of the body, laziness
• Pain and stiffness in the thigh	• Burning sensation in shoulder	• Excess saliva and mucus Excessive excretion of excreta
• Paraplegia	• Excessive temperature, excessive sweating	• Loss of strength
• Prolapsed rectum	• Fetid odour of the body	• Indigestion
• Pain in scrotum, stiffness in penis, groin, pelvic area	• Cracking pain in the body	• Phlegm accumulated in the vicinity of heart and throat
• Diarrhea	• Sloughing of the blood	• Hardening of vessels
• Lameness, dwarfism	• Burning sensation of the skin, cracking of the skin, itching of the skin, urtecaria	• Goiter
• Stiffness of back, of neck	• Red vesicle	• Obesity
• Pain in chest, in abdomen	• Tendency to bleed	• Suppression of digestive power.
• Trouble in thoracic movement (lung movement)	• Blue moles	• Urtecaria
• Atrophy of arm	• Herpes	
• Hoarseness in voice		

Diseases of mover (*vata*)	Diseases of transformer (*pitta*)	Diseases of binder (*kapha*)
• Pain in jaw, lips, eyes, teeth, earaches	• Jaundice (yellowish colouration of eyes, urine and feces)	• Whiteness of urine and feces.
• Astringent taste in the mouth, dryness of mouth	• Bitter taste in mouth	
• Hard of hearing, deafness	• Fetid odour of mouth	
• Cataract, pain in eyes	• Excessive thirst	
• Pain in temporal and frontal regions	• Conjunctivitis	
• Headache	• Inflammation of the penis	
• Dandruff	• Hemorrhage	
• Facial paralysis	• Greenish and yellowish colouration of eyes, urine and feces	
• Fainting, giddiness, tremour, yawning, hiccups		
• Delirium		
• Insomnia		
• Unstable mentality		

medicinal diet *triphala*

Triphala (or three fruits) is a combination of three herbal fruits. They are *amla (phyllanthus emblica), harad (Terminalia chebula)* and *behada (Terminalia belerica)*.

This combination is light and dry. It has five of the six tastes: sweet, sour, pungent, bitter and astringent. By virtue of having these tastes, *triphala* controls food cravings.

- It is cooling in potency and its post digestive effect is sweet.

- It balances all the three *doshas*. It rejuvenates all the bodily tissues and clears all the channels (*srotas*). It is used as a mild laxative, which is not habit forming. It relieves chronic constipation and strengthens the gastrointestinal tract. It cleanses the body of accumulated wastes. According to Ayurveda it digests the toxins (*ama*) from the body, at the same time nourishing the tissues. It improves digestion and assimilation. It is used as a part of daily routine when the body shows signs of sluggishness, indigestion or flatulence.

- It is anti- inflammatory, anti-viral and has rejuvenating qualities.

- It clears the lungs of mucus and strengthens the respiratory channels.

- It is used to treat skin inflammations, boils and other skin conditions like acne and boils.

- It is used as a mouthwash. It cures bleeding gums.

- It is used as an infusion or eyewash to keep the eyes healthy and is also used in conditions of eye inflammations, conjunctivitis or sties etc.

- *Triphala* is a complete detoxification preparation for the whole system.

- *Triphala* is also an elixir. It can be taken every day (3 to 5 gms) with milk, clarified butter (for *vata* and *pitta* people) or honey (for *kapha* people). It nourishes and raises general immunity of the body.

sacred healing plant *tulsi*/basil

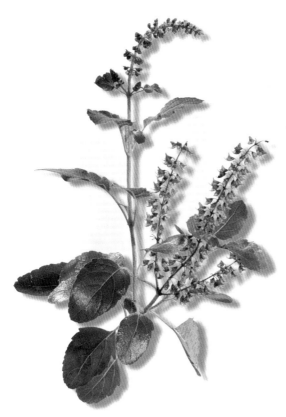

Tulsi: Basil, (*Ocimum sanctum*) is a useful plant to have at home.

It is a greatly valued herb in Ayurveda. *Tulsi* is hot, pungent, light, dry, rough, sharp and subtle. The post-digestive effect of *tulsi* is pungent. All parts of the plant – the root, stem, leaves, flower and seeds are used for medicinal purposes. They can be dried and kept in a powdered form. Fresh juice of *tulsi* leaves is particularly effective as a preventive and curative medicine. *Tulsi* is antibacterial, antiviral and anti fungal. It is also anti-inflammatory. However, it is contraindicated during pregnancy (being hot), for lactating mothers (it decreases breast milk) and for women trying to conceive.

According to Ayurveda, *tulsi* cures coughs hiccups, breathing problems, backaches and intestinal worms. It also removes all kinds of bad odours from the body as well as from food.

It acts directly on *prana* (vital breath) carrying, blood carrying and *rasa* carrying channels. It helps in digesting *ama* and is curative of most of the phlegmatic disorders of the throat, mouth, lungs and the upper respiratory tract. It is used in treatment of tuberculosis, leprosy and many other difficult skin conditions.

Uses

▶ The fresh juice of *tulsi* leaves (one teaspoon) and honey (one teaspoon) can be mixed together and consumed slowly. It removes mucus from the tongue, throat and chest. It prevents phlegm from entering the lungs, however, if the lungs are already affected, it clears the phlegm from the lungs.

▶ Fresh leaves of *tulsi* (ten) and five black peppercorns *(kali mirch)*, boiled in a glass of water for 10 minutes can be sipped warm twice a day. This decoction contains fevers, and is especially effective in malarial fever.

▶ Rubbing the juice of *tulsi* leaves relieves the pain and sting of an insect bite or any poisonous bite. It also helps in treating skin infections.

▶ The juice of *tulsi* leaves and honey mixed together stops vomiting in children.

▶ A few drops of juice of *tulsi* leaves can be used to alleviate earaches.

▶ A decoction of all parts of the plant is very useful in for influenza and common colds. The juice of *tulsi* leaves with equal amounts of ginger juice and honey cures coughs and colds, but should not be given for dry coughs.

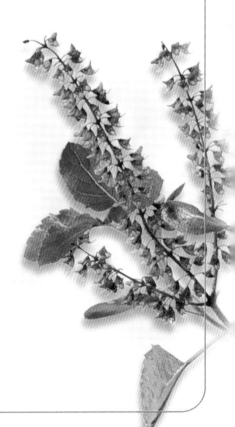

▶ A powder of the dry *tulsi* leaves with honey, taken twice a day proves beneficial in diabetic conditions.

▶ Apart from medicinal and culinary aspects, *tulsi* also has a spiritual aspect for many Indian households. It is considered sacred, as it has a purifying effect on the mind and body as well as on its' surroundings.

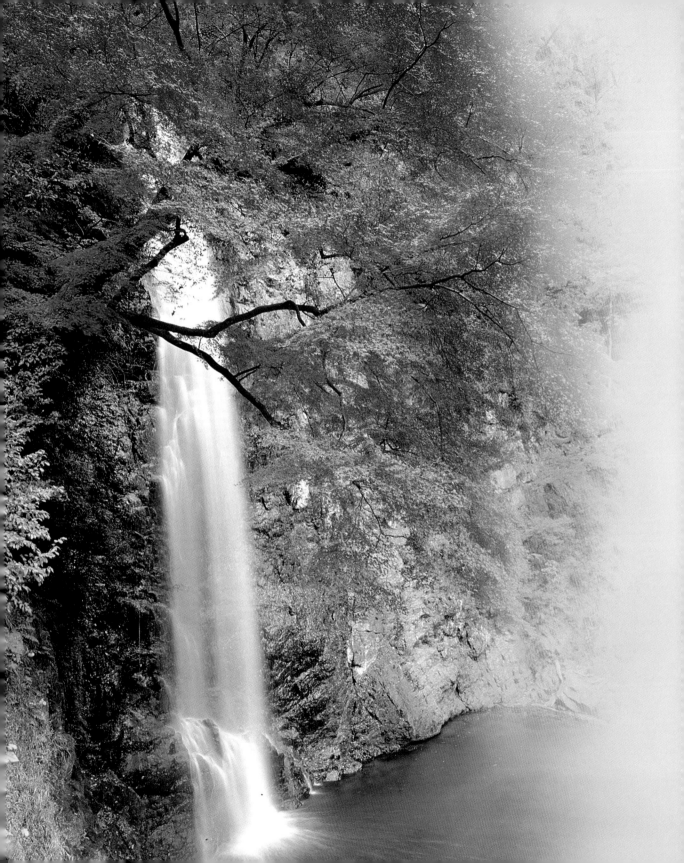

conclusion:
the ayurvedic way

~

A Few Precautions

Ayurveda is a theory of felt body, of sensate matter and of health and disease in a person. Thus living with Ayurveda, ideally, should be a natural agenda for one and all. However, this is not the case. The development of science has brought about serious confusion regarding this agenda. The fundamentals of Ayurveda are radically different from the medical theory based on modern science. It is commonly believed that modern science on the one hand and Ayurveda on the other are working at crossroads. Confusion occurs because the connection between sensate matter and insensate matter is not obvious and clear. The matter is the same, though theorizations about the sensate and insensate aspect of matter in Ayurveda and in science respectively differs and often is pitched against each other. This shows not only in debatable medical practices of the two but also in everyday contentious nutritional and hygiene practices promoted by the two. It is here that some amount of cautious consideration is required.

In Ayurveda, there is scope for the effect of insensate matter on the person through the notion of the *prabhava* (powers) of substances. Modern medical knowledge on the other hand has no place for sensate matter. However, modern medical practice does take recourse to sensate matter in a theoretically *ad hoc* manner based on the acceptance of some of the traditional practices of food and hygiene. Thus downward integration of Ayurvedic and modern knowledge is possible and plausible whereas upward integration of modern medicine and Ayurveda is not that natural.

Whatever be the current state of acculturation between Ayurveda and modern science, one point can be emphatically made – as far as diet and hygiene go Ayurveda has a clear theoretical edge over modern science. Since the common man's acceptance of Ayurvedic medicines is not yet complete, doubts range from skepticism to forthright rejection. It is ironic that only those Ayurvedic drugs that are found to be effective according to biomedical criteria become part of the mainstream medicine.

A modern lifestyle has affected traditional Ayurvedic practices on account of changes in time. Not only have hordes of new material products (of industrial origin) come into use by man, but also several traditions of food and hygiene practices have come face to face because of the blending of different cultures. Substances in use by different cultures and in different regions have become globally available. Products like chocolates, coffee, tea etc. can nonetheless be accommodated within Ayurvedic theory since they can be examined and evaluated as sensate matter. But there is a need to characterize many new edible products in accordance with Ayurvedic theory. This is true even for a variety of herbal products originating from different regions. Such a task needs to be addressed for Ayurveda to become a way of life in modern times.

In the wake of several alternative modern proposals on nutrition that seem attractive today, there is a need to comparatively evaluate the approach of Ayurveda. For example, several dietary prescriptions are available; there is a high protein diet, a rainbow diet, a diet for diabetics, a diet for those with heart ailments, weight loss diets and so on. All these proposals cater to specific nutritional requirements that usually arise in adverse situations of the body. It is only for specific needs that people turn to these diets. A diet under normal circumstances for all ages and requirements is not comprehensively addressed by these proposals. They deal with restrictive situations. Ayurveda, on the other hand, addresses dietetics in a comprehensive way catering to all situations of body – right from childhood to old age; from normal to abnormal conditions of body, and from different body types to different time regimens.

The first step in living in accordance with Ayurveda is understanding the three vitalities (*doshas*) – mover, transformer and binder. Not only will one's own body get better understood with these concepts in terms of knowing the basic constitution of the body, but the desirable/undesirable effects of diet/drugs can be be rationally understood. It is important to cross-check the constitution of one's own body from an experienced Ayurvedic practitioner. It is also important to accurately know one's body constitution since reasoning in Ayurveda crucially depends on it. It needs to be stressed that the concept of vitalities characterizes functional disposition of the body as well as dysfunctionality in the body. These concepts are central to Ayurveda and any one who can intuit and reason with them is a master of Ayurveda!

Once the constitution of the body is securely and authentically known, it is easy to interpret the effect of various time-cycles on the body as time cycles directly affect the functional aspect of the body or vitalities. Designing a healthy diet for a particular person thus becomes possible and easily understandable. We become intelligently equipped to understand the response of the body to environmental changes. Though these effects can be overlooked in reckless living without immediate adverse effects but in the long run these effects are very significant for the upkeep of person in good spirit and healthy body. Disciplined living is the key to freedom from chronic and debilitating diseases. The body varies with and responds to different time cycles; being sensitive to these changes helps navigate the body intelligently with little effort. Understanding environmental effects in terms of three vitalities is the second step in intelligent living with Ayurveda. The situation, receptivity and vulnerability of the body at any particular time of the day, week, month, season and epoch in life is understood through the knowledge of body constitution and environment.

Understanding the material substances that are normally used as food in terms of sensate properties is the third step in living with Ayurveda. Ayurveda helps in understanding the sensate characteristics of different kinds of edible substances. It is these sensate characteristics that in turn help us understand effect of these substances on the body. Any imbalance in the body in terms of increase or decrease in the three vitalities can be corrected with the help of a particular diet or specific food substance. This is in addition to the knowledge which Ayurveda provides as to how different edible substances build various tissues of the body. The sensate character or attributes of matter directly affect vitalities, which themselves are bundles of sensate attributes of matter. Similar qualities accentuate one another, wheras dissimilar qualities suppress each other. This is a fundamental causal principle employed by Ayurveda. After the constitution of the body is determined and environmental effects are understood, if nourishing features of edible substances are understood as well, much of what is involved in living with Ayurveda is accomplished.

Some edible substances are not taken regularly, but have useful applications as drugs in case of illness. Any edible substance can either act as food that nourishes the organism, medicine that balances the organism or as poison that disturbs the organism. Many common illnesses can be handled with the help of ordinarily available natural substances. Ayurveda helps identify the use of these common substances for common ailments. Any complications regarding diseases need to be strictly handled by experts. This is because actual complications in the body are indeed complex and the strategies to handle them are doubly complex. Though these very same principles are used for diagnostics and therapeutics, they are used with a sophisticated grasp of interaction among them in a particular body with multiple fault lines.

Ayurveda does not have standard drugs like allopathic formularies. Industrially mass produced Ayurvedic drugs overlook particularities characterizing any serious imbalance in a specific body. One unique feature of Ayurveda is the minute attention given to the particularities of disease differing from body to body and condition to condition. Further, self-prescribed drugs can backfire if they are not for short-term common ailments. All this needs to be kept in mind while attending to illnesses. It is a common error to take surface symptoms for deep-seated diseases that cause those symptoms. Please consult expert practitioners while venturing into self-medication for serious diseases.

Ayurveda regards cognitive misdemeanour (*prajnaparadha*) as the primary cause of all illnesses. Not being able to understand how to live with Ayurveda is one such cognitive failure. Such a lapse leads to counter productive habits of bodily conduct, including the intake of wrong substances, bad excretion, an irregular and mindless routine. Prolonged fear, anxiety, aggression, tension, longing, and fatigue are sure signs of developing malfunctions in the body and an imbalanced person.

The mind is a charioteer of the body. If the mind develops bad habits, the body is left to mend on its own without an anchor or a rudder. A rudderless body sinks into the abyss of one illness after another. The *Caraka Samhita* says that, 'Leaving aside all other things, the body is to be protected with great care; for, in its absence, all other activities (of human beings) cease to exist.' Living with Ayurveda amounts to not letting the body and mind drift mindlessly such that it is of little use to itself and to others. Ayurveda provides a holistic path to intelligent living, making perfect health a matter of choice.

references

Bhishagracharya, Sri Satyapala, 'Vrddha Jivaka,' *Kasyapa Samhita*, 4th edition.
Chaukhamba Sanskrit Sansthan. Varanasi, 1994.

Bhishagratana, Kaviraj Kunjalal (Ed), *Susruta Samhita*. Chaukhamba Sanskrit Sansthan. Varanasi. 1981.

Dash, Vaidya Bhagwan and Lalitesh Kashyap (Eds), *Five Specialized Therapies of Ayurveda, Pancakarma: Based on Ayurveda Saukhyam of Todarananda*. Vedams Books. Delhi. 1992.

Misra, Sri Brahma Sankara and Sri Rupalalji Vaisya (Eds), *The Bravaprakasa I-II*.
Chaukhamba Sanskrit Sansthan. Varanasi. 1969.

Murthy, Srikantha K.R. *Vagbhatta, Astanga (Sangra) Hrdayam*. Krishnadas Academy. Varanasi. 1996.

Sharma, R.K. and Vaidya Bhagwan Dash (Trs), *Agnivesa's Caraka Samhita: Text with Critical Exposition Based on Cakrapani Datta's Dipika*. Chaukhamba Sanskrit Sansthan, vol. XCIV. Varanasi. 2002.

The Ayurvedic Formulary of India, Part I, Second edition. Controller of Publication. Delhi. 2003.

The Ayurvedic Formulary of India, Part II. Controller of Publication. Delhi. 2000.

glossary

Abhyanga: Morning massage

Adanaka: Acquisition time

Adhipati marma: First vital point (the crown of the head)

Agni (also *tejas*): Fire

Ahara: Food

Ajwain: Carom seeds or Bishop's weed

Akasa: Space

Alocakagni: Sight fires

Ama: Waste (undigested or toxic matter present in the body)

Amala: Sour taste

Amlaki: (*Emblica officinalis*) Indian gooseberry

Anubhava: Experience

Apa: Water

Apana vayu: Air responsible for evacuation from the body

Atman: Self

Ayus: All aspects pertaining to personhood

Babul: (*Acacia arabica*) Acacia

Bael: (*Aegle marmelos*) Indian bael fruit

Bala taila: Head massage with a cloth soaked in oil

Bhrajakagni: Absorption fire

Cakra: Wheel

Chana: Chickpeas

Dalchini: Cinnamon

Desa: The state of health and the digestive capacity of a person

Dhania: Coriander

Dhara: Pouring of oil or buttermilk on the body, or specific body parts

Dhatus: The vital tissue elements

Dosha: Fault prone vitality

Dravya: Substance

Elaichi: Cardamom

Gharsana: Dry friction massage

Ghee: Clarified butter

Gud: Jaggery

Guna: Indicator of the material composition of a substance

Haldi: Turmeric

Haritaki: (*Harad, Terminalia chebula*) Indian gallnut

Heeng: Asafoetida

Indriya: Sense organs

Jaiphal: Nutmeg

Jataragni: Digestive fire

Jeera: Black cumin

Kala: Time periods (time of day or night, season etc.)

Kali mirch: Black pepper

Kapha: Binder

Kasaya: Astringent taste

Kattu: Pungent taste

Kesar: Saffron

Kosha: Sheath enclosing the self (*atman*)

Lassi: Yogurt drink

Lavana: Salty taste

Lavanga: Clove

Lepam: The application of herbal paste

Madhura: Sweet taste

Mala: Waste matter

Manas: The heart-mind

Marma: The point at which ligaments, bones, muscle tissues and joints meet

Masur: Red lentil

Matra: Quantity of food (*atimatra* refers to over eating; *hinamatra* refers to under eating)

Methi: Fenugreek

Misri: Crystal sugar

Mung: Green gram

Nasya: application of oil inside the nostrils (part of *pancakarma* therapy. See below)

Neem: (*Azadirachta indica*) Indian neem

Ojas: Subtle spiritual energy, opposite of *ama*

Pakvasaya: Colon

Pancakama: Preventive and curative therapeutic tool consisting of *vamana* (drugs given to induce vomiting), *virecana* (therapeutic purgation) *basti* (medicated enemas) *nasya* (nasal

medication) and *rakta moksana* (blood letting)

Panca mahabhutas: Five elements

Pichu: Tamping of *marmas*

Pippali: (*Piper longum Linn*) long pepper

Pitta: Transformer

Prabhava: Power

Prakriti: The constitution of a person

Prana vayu: Air connected with activities of the mind

Pranayama: Observing and controlling vital breath

Prayatna: Action

Prithvi: Earth

Rajma: Kidney beans

Ranjakagni: Metabolic fire

Rasa: Flavour or taste

Ritu: Season(*Sisira*: later winter; *Vasanta*: spring; *Grisma*: summer; *Varsa*: rainy; *Hemanta*: early winter)

Sadhakagni: Apparitional fire

Samskara: Disposition of a person

Sarada purnima: Full moon

Sarira: Body

Sattva gunas: Quintessential qualities

Saunf: Fennel seeds

Saunth: Dry ginger powder

Sharbat: Cooling drink made from fruit and herbs

Sikha: Whirl where the hair parts on the head

Sirobasti: Keeping oil on the head contained by a cap

Sirovecana: Elimination of *doshas* from the head

Snehan: Oileation

Srota: Bodily channel

Surya namaskar: Sun salutation

Svedana: Sweat

Tikta: Bitter and hot

Til: Sesame

Trikatu: A preparation containing the fruits of black pepper, long pepper and rhizomes of ginger

Triphala: The three fruits of Ayurveda: amlaki (*Emblica officinalis*), haritaki (*Terminalia chebula*) and bibhitaki (*Terminalia belerica*)

Tulsi: (*Ocimum sanctum*) Basil

Ubtana: Herbal paste massage

Upayoga vyavasta: Dietetic rules

Upyoktrin: Individual dietary habits

Urad: Black gram

Utsepa marma: Temporal lobe

Vaca: Calamus

Vata: Mover

Vayu: Air

Vikriti: Imbalance

Vipaka: Aftertaste

Viruddha ahara: Incompatible foods

Virya: Heating or cooling potential

Visargakala: Parting time

Yajna: Fire sacrifice

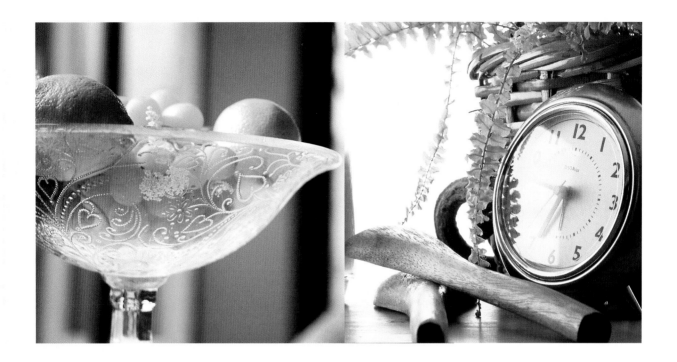

ISBN: 81-7436-361-0

© Roli & Janssen BV 2005
Published in India by Roli Books
in arrangement with Roli & Janssen BV
M-75, Greater Kailash-II (Market)
New Delhi-110 048, India.
Phones: ++91-11-29212271, 29212782,
Fax: ++91-11-29217185
Email: roli@vsnl.com, Website: rolibooks.com

Editor: Nandita Jaishankar
Design: Sneha Pamneja
Page layout: Kumar Raman
Photographs: Roli Collection

Printed and bound at Singapore

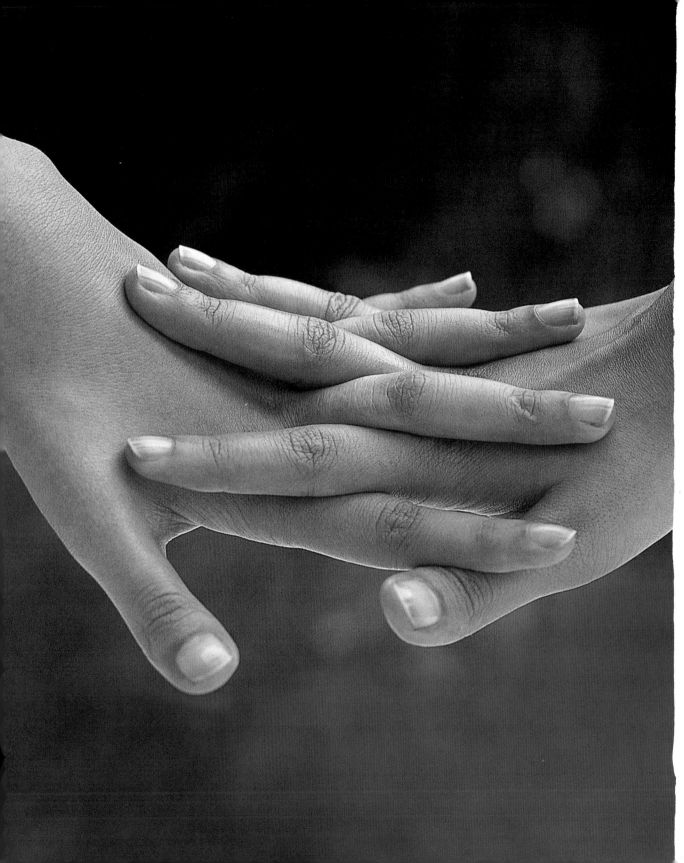